MIND *to* MOUTH

MIND *to* MOUTH

A Busy Chick's Guide to Mindful Mealtime Moments

HEATHER SEARS

Kensho Press
Boston, MA

Published in 2017 by Kensho Press
Printed in the United States of America
ISBN: 978-0-9993043-0-3
Library of Congress Control Number: 2017915939
Kensho Press, Boston, MA

Cover design by Fusion Creative Works
Interior design by Kiran Spees

The author is not affiliated with, nor did she receive any compensation from, Habit, Nestlé, or Whole Foods. The words and
content provided in this book are not intended and should not be
construed as medical advice. If readers have a medical concern,
they should consult with an appropriately licensed medical
professional. Never disregard professional medical advice or delay
in seeking it because of something you have read in this book.

Breathe. Taste. Savor. Smile.

—Heather Sears

Contents

Part II: Mouth

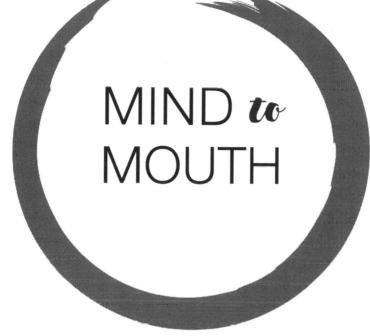

A Day in the Life of a Mindful Busy Chick

Workday Lunch

- Create a mindful food space.

- Listen to your tummy; eat at your own pace and not the pace of the office.

- Remove distractions; if in a crunch, set a timer and stay screen-free until it goes off.

In the Car

- Eat only at stoplights.

- Keep your eyes on the road.

- If kids are in the back, breathe; don't yell.

At the Bar

- With wine, chill; let your mind be still.

- Notice noise: find a quiet spot to maximize flavor.

- Lean in to the conversation, and savor.

Famished Fam

- Serve food on small, separate plates.

- Increase variety to increase attention and enjoyment.

- Play music from the meal's country of origin to emphasize ethnic taste.

Shopping Mission

- Before shopping, plan.

- While shopping, breathe.

- After shopping, practice self-kindness by putting your feet up and enjoying a rest!

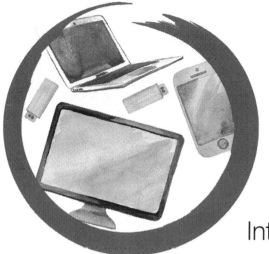

Introduction

Too Busy to Swallow

Growing up, I could often be found sitting bare-foot at the family table, long hair uncombed, eating fresh, homemade yogurt. My mom grew alfalfa sprouts on the counter. The tomatoes and cucumbers came from the garden. And we regularly visited the health food co-op for bulk grains and carob treats. This was way before it was trendy—back when chia seeds were used in chia pets, not puddings. My mom was a beautiful mix of earthy artist and self-educated sophis-tication, and she taught me what it meant to nourish myself with real food.

Her influence led me to other forms of nourishment too. In a moment of curiosity one day while I was in high school, I picked up one of my mom's books about meditation. I started attending weekly meditation sessions with her and developed a daily practice of my own, which helped calm my turbulent teenage thoughts and moody emotions. In those early years, I was training my attention and cultivating inner stillness late into the night.

Fast forward to today. I'm now an urban mom who works in the always-on world of digital media. Life seems to have gotten progressively denser: multichannel work demands, childcare and mommy duties, household management, trying to squeeze in a workout (often unsuccessfully), planning and prepping every meal. Rinse. Repeat. Repeat.

The modern treadmill.

For years, I rushed through day after day as I tried to check every item off my growing to-do list. This pace sped up when I was working from home with my son in preschool, intensely multitasking to get work finished before pick-up time. And then I started choking.

I would be triple-tasking as usual while eating my lunch at the counter or even while walking to the table. The food would get caught in my throat and just not go down. I would have to sit very still for what felt like an eternity, hacking away, waiting for my throat to clear so I could swallow.

This happened repeatedly. At the same time, I was making progressively less healthy, more impulsive and convenient food choices for my family and myself, serving a diet of microwaved mush and takeout.

I'm part country girl—tied to the land, drawn to farm-fresh food and home cooking—and part city chick, happy to embrace tech and packaged time-savers that help me get it all done. But the woes of modern life had taken over; I felt like I'd lost a part of myself. I didn't feel like me. While I still valued and craved nourishing, delicious mealtime experiences, I was focused on getting each gotta-do done and had lost the sparks of inspiration that in the past drove the creation of meals filled with flavor, warmth, and contentment: the food that restored and revived me. I was cooking and eating but not at all satisfied.

This had become a pattern, and something had to change. While I wanted to blame someone or something else, namely my cats for not intervening when they saw me making poor choices, I realized that what I needed to change was me.

So, what exactly was going on here? I knew how to make healthy food choices. My mom had given me many lessons about reading food labels: that's why only the best chocolate will do! I knew how to cook, from time spent in the family kitchen and in more formal culinary school classes, and I enjoyed it. I also loved food. I'd tasted my way around the globe, and had taken over 30 food-focused trips to France, Italy, and Switzerland. With all this attention to the subject, I *thought* I was self-aware. But I was doing none of the things I knew to do.

So, I started observing and asking questions. I watched my head and heart and behavior in the context of mealtimes and I began researching. I looked into societal trends, our eating environment, and food marketing.

I harkened back to my university days as an Asian Studies major and dug into ancient books about meditation and mindfulness; reviewed food psychology and gastrophysics research; and interviewed corporate executives, chefs, and mindfulness experts. I tapped into my professional marketing knowledge and existing meditation practice. I drank a lot of wine and coffee while discussing the topic with girlfriends. They were facing similar challenges.

This book shares my journey—my struggles and my questions, my discoveries, and the solution that worked for me, one based on ancient wisdom combined with modern data, and grounded in fun, practical ideas for how you can apply it within your active life. Let's face it: our lives don't slow down just because we start choking or need to lose weight or want more zen during dinnertime. But as busy as we are, we can still make changes that allow us to start nourishing ourselves again, or maybe even for the first time.

And I've learned that it begins with being mindful.

Mindfulness brings so many benefits, and it's simple once we know how to do it and start to notice differences, pay attention to new things, and get interested in what's around us. In the pages ahead, I'll give you tips on how to do this, and share interesting data about environmental triggers, mental blind spots, and contextual influences, all of which will help you start noticing things you may have overlooked before. This will help you begin to create great meals with intention.

After reading, practicing, and journaling your way through this book, you will have a working knowledge of mindfulness and a simple practice to get you started; you will be more aware of and equipped to respond to the forces you are up against on your mealtime journey; and you will have a deeper appreciation for yourself and your innate ability to create any mealtime outcome you desire.

That's what I experienced, and what I hope for you. This exploration has been a gift, and I want to share it. And also, because through this process, I discovered how many subliminal influences we must contend with. We need presence of mind if we are to make healthy choices regarding food and make our experiences with the food we eat satisfyingly our own.

To get there, I promise you won't need to pull out your old college textbooks or even go to a yoga studio (unless you want to). These pages draw upon my research, interviews, and decades-long practice of mindfulness and meditation, and put it all together in a way you can use, starting right now.

Here are three key takeaways:

It's them. It's me. If not now, when?

It's them. There are a number of surprising, practically invisible, coming-from-all-directions external influences and mixed messages that impact our mealtime behavior and enjoyment. These stem from many things, including environmental sources and the use of digital devices.

It's me. We experience many nonlinear and transient internal moments of assessment, intent, and decision on our journey to mealtime outcomes. Our minds create our meal experiences, and it starts way before the first bite. We have assumptions and habits that drive our actions and direct our attention. Our attitudes are trained to be expectant and impulsive these days.

If not now, when? We must practice mindfulness in real time. Meditation is very helpful, but it's not the main event—each moment presents an opportunity to create our experience if we are interested enough to notice. While it takes a little nudge to your attention to remember to be present in the moment, it is not difficult. It is a skill that can be easily learned, and success can be tasted immediately.

All this led me to the realization that conscious, mindful micro-moments while on my food-consumption journey were the answer to my problems. *How* we plan, shop, and prepare our meals greatly impacts what we put in our mouths. Our state of being during the many moments of our journey can make the difference between a rushed, crappy meal that we don't even notice we are eating and a wholesome, nourishing, tasty meal that was prepared efficiently and with grace.

Luckily, this pivot in approach is not one more thing to *do*. Because seriously, who has more time in the day? It's an inner shift.

Once I made this shift to a more mindful state of being, I noticed changes that brought surprising but pleasant results: I have more time, joy, space for kindness, and more money in my pocket. I have less anxiety, and I dropped excess weight.

I saved time by reshaping my attitude and approach to planning meals and shopping, by using digital technology to support my needs, and by developing a conscious relationship with my phone, email inbox, and social media accounts. I stopped compulsively checking all digital channels, which has given me at least 50 hours back daily. Okay, maybe not 50, but it feels like 50!

The joy I experience during mealtime has increased because I consciously appreciate my surroundings and actually taste my food, even on those rare occasions when I eat with my phone nearby. It's still a process, and it's important to recognize that life happens, and we won't always be 100 percent present. As I became more aware of the food I was eating and its various tastes and textures, I developed new preferences in coffee, water, apples, chocolate, and pizza. And, I can now tell you exactly how I like my oatmeal prepared. I have also identified a few foods that don't suit me anymore.

More joy led to more space for kindness in my heart and, hence, my meals. When I slowed down what was going on in my head, there was an immediate opening of my heart. Increased kindness to myself translated to more kindness to my family. I say yes more: to a cup of tea and piece of cake at 4:00 p.m., to my son's request to make Play-Doh fantasy worlds on the kitchen floor while I'm cooking, to eating breakfast as a picnic in front of the fireplace on cold winter days. The kindness and openheartedness replaced some habitual resistance and inner criticizing. Now we have more togetherness and less irritation.

And if all that wasn't enough, we spend less on food now. All the preplanning, prep, and choosing foods that better suit us reduced our takeout, delivery, and grocery expenses. When I reviewed our accounts, we decreased costs by 14–24 percent!

I lost the guilt I used to feel over our food spending, and along with it, the anxiety I used to feel when preparing meals. The sometimes grumpy predinner behavior of my family did not change—I did. And my approach to serving meals has evolved along the way. As it has changed, my son's attitude has too. He seems to complain less, and as any mom can tell you, that's a big stress relief.

I've cleansed my kitchen of clutter—and expired spices, vitamins, and almond milk. It's now a welcoming, calming space for creating mealtime experiences that satisfy everyone at our table.

Now that I'm better in touch with my feelings and sense of hunger and satisfaction, I've switched up how much and when I eat. I also switched my fitness practice because I'm more aware of what works best for me given my constraints. I dropped some weight and feel at ease, happy. Referring to a picture taken recently, my husband actually said that I looked like Jennifer Aniston! And while I don't believe that I look like her, I know I glow like she does because I feel great, and great shows.

Now I've got a homemade green smoothie groove goin' on, and I make many more satisfying, personalized food choices for my family and me.

I used to think I didn't have time to cook healthy meals, but now I do so weekly. And btw, I take a high-low approach to eating where I'm hands-on where it counts for me and use other options for the rest: frozen pizza alongside fresh salad with apples and pinot noir, homemade curried squash soup with store-bought naan, freshly baked healthy breakfast cookies and Starbucks coffee, premade mac and cheese with fresh-roasted chicken. Mindfulness helps me make choices I feel good about, and it helps me make these choices efficiently.

This is **A B**usy **C**hick's approach to mindful mealtimes. It is a way of being. A practice of presence and awareness. It's designed to help you consciously reshape your choices and perspectives in real time. And it's as easy as ABC.

When I want to ground myself in mindful presence, in the Now, I do what I call an ABC check-in. You can do them too. In a check-in, we simply focus on **At**tention to the present moment; **Breathing,** to center the mind and move from our chattering narrative to calmly and directly experience life as it is; and **C**uriosity, which causes us to tune in to ourselves and explore our environment, to get to know what is happening in our mind, body, and heart as well as our surroundings.

I'll go into more detail about the ABC check-ins in chapter 2. Just be aware of them for now because mindfulness allows us to disrupt preprogrammed narratives and inputs and allows us to consciously choose our responses to incoming information based on new awareness.

Repeating these ABC moments many times as we plan, shop, prepare, and eat builds an intimate understanding of ourselves through our skillful observation. The repetition also builds mind muscle memory that leads to heightened awareness and conscious choices becoming natural habits over time.

So, what type of mealtime experience do you want to create, and how do you want to feel along the way to creating it? You will develop your own food groove. Each of our journeys unfolds in unique, personal ways, but we're all influenced by many of the same factors, and we can all benefit from what I've discovered.

Each moment on your journey, whether you are on the go and trying to figure out dinner or at the holiday table with in-laws, holds potential for lighthearted ease, profound appreciation, and great contentment. By increasing your knowledge of mealtime influencers and practicing mindful ABCs, you can enter into the present moment and taste the joy that is waiting for you.

And joy tastes great, kind of like jelly beans on a sunny day.

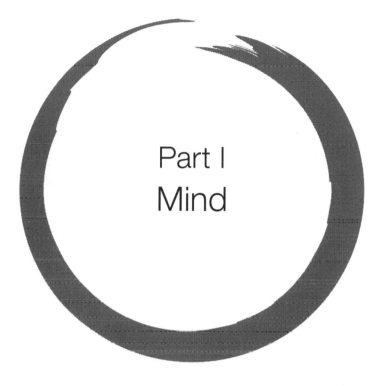

Part I
Mind

1

Too Busy to Taste

When I dug into the research, I found many things that didn't surprise me. Today, women cook less at home. It is estimated we eat 20 percent of our meals in the car.[1] Our addiction to smartphones is training us to have shorter attention spans. Unhealthy food is omnipresent and can be summoned with a frictionless slide and tap of a finger. Of course, we already know all this.

Here's what did surprise me: The magnitude of our exhausting everyday-athon is shifting food consumption at a macro level and creating new industries to serve our needs. The social-mobile foodscape is directly correlated to weight gain. Our identities and expectation-driven attitudes impact our food choice. There is a plethora of nearly invisible environmental factors that influence our consumption behavior and enjoyment. And, businesses are unlocking detailed data and gaining insights into our intentions and actions on a moment-to-moment basis and are using this information to get their products in our mouths.

I also discovered that researchers have estimated that we have approximately 60,000 thoughts per day![2] And, over 80 percent of our thoughts are supposedly repeated from day to day and are negative.[3] Just like our unconscious food decisions, many of our thoughts are running in the background repeating a narrative that may be influencing our lives in ways differently than we would prefer.

We're also not aware of how many food-related decisions we make. Researchers have found that we make around 200 more food decisions a day than we think we do! Many of these are "automatic" food choices, when we mindlessly eat without considering what, where, when, or how much food we're selecting and consuming. This lack of awareness can lead to overconsumption and weight gain.[4]

We may not be aware of our choices, but data-savvy businesses are. We can't hide our food habits from them. Our smartphones track our location data, and companies can gain access to this data and combine it with our search, social, app-use, and shopping data to create detailed profiles of our lifestyles and habits. They can predict our intentions and see our actions nearly in real time.

Companies are also using neuromarketing techniques to study the human brain's responses to marketing stimuli and to improve their tactics. Neuromarketing impacts behavior that is largely automatic, emotional, and outside our conscious awareness. Examples include utilizing eye-tracking studies that determine what shelf placement will most likely lead to a product purchase, organizing supermarket shelving color and lighting to optimize sales,[5] and even focusing the viewer on ad content by positioning babies to look directly at the product being advertised.[6] These businesses know us better than we know ourselves, and they use this knowledge to reach and influence us with their marketing.

Digital marketing and retail food setups aren't the only environmental factors influencing what, when, and how much we eat. Where we eat plays a big role too.

More than ever, we're now eating away from home. In 2015 Americans started spending more money at bars and restaurants than on groceries.[7] This is too bad because cooking at home is directly correlated with weighing less—not surprising since portion sizes in restaurants have doubled and even tripled in the last two decades.[8]

There is a mountain of research about how the kitchen and dining environment (plateware, glass-ware, cutlery, sound, lighting, the amount of clutter, etc.) influence how much we eat and the enjoyment we feel during a meal. In one study, people took and ate 31 percent more food as a result of having been given an exaggerated environmental cue (such as a large bowl). Of those studied, 21 percent denied having eaten more, 75 percent attributed eating more to other reasons (such as hunger), and only 4 percent attributed their increased consumption to the cue.[9] "We think we're smarter than the environment around us," Professor Brian Wansink, director of the Food and Brand Lab at Cornell University, states. "That's why these external cues are so powerful." We may be unaware that they are impacting our actions, yet they clearly influence us deeply.[10]

When we do eat at home, we have more control over external cues like portion and plate size, but even if we are aware of these, the reality of our home life often presents further challenges. The modern dinner table has been transformed. The completely home-cooked-by-mom meal, identically served on each plate with only the TV on in the background, is on the way out.

Now each person may have personalized plates of food based on his or her diet-of-the-day preferences served with a mobile phone on the side and fitness tracker on the wrist.

This happens at my table. I eat differently than my husband and son. It's not just our difference of opinion on the tastiness of mushrooms and tomatoes ("poisonous fruit," says my husband); we are each aware of how different foods function in our bodies and want to optimize our meals. And while we do not have any screens or tech at our table, they are certainly only a few steps away.

"Flexitarian" diets, where people roll between different styles of eating within the day and week, are growing in popularity. We may eat paleo during the day and switch to gluten-free at night. We may eat local for a week and then just vegetarian. People are experimenting with different diet styles by customizing bits and pieces of their meals.[11] This may be due in part to the large amount of somewhat confusing and contradictory data about different diets. We get curious and want to test out various things.

It's clear that modern mealtimes bear little resemblance to the traditional family meals many of us enjoyed growing up.

Dining on Digital

Those smartphones so often lying next to our plates play an outsize role in our changing eating experience. In our busy world, we're often consuming more than food at our tables; we are constantly ingesting digital data, and it's beginning to give us bellyaches.

The ever-growing amount of content is staggering. Users post more than 100 million photos on Instagram and Twitter every day. Add this to the modern overwhelm list. Lorena Jones, VP of Ten Speed Press, describes it well: "That great blossoming of so much content was wonderful—until it was totally oppressive and overwhelming and hard to get through. There was no filter; you became the filter."[12]

The food information we filter from digital media is believed to influence over 70 percent of the food eaten in American households.[13] Food triggers our pleasure response.

Receiving texts and social media "likes," along with other forms of online engagement, releases dopamine, which provides the same addictive, feel-good jolt as sex.[14] No wonder we keep our phones within arm's reach 24/7. The neuroplasticity of our brains (the process by which the brain changes in response to experience) trains us to look for these pings of pleasure. That's why we reactively keep checking—a lot. On average, people check their phones 150 times per day.[15] That means we're looking at our screens every 6.4 minutes during waking hours!

We live in an expectation economy where we expect to have information at our fingertips and on our smartphones, and instant task completion is the name of the game. And by instant, I mean instant: 53 percent of mobile users now abandon sites that take longer than three seconds to load.[16] And in this new reality, we have to ask: Is instant gratification making us perpetually impatient, and are ever-present images of food making us perpetually hungry?

You may have noticed the glorious images of food everywhere you look online. Pinterest's Food and Drink category had 13 billion saved ideas between January and November of 2016.[17] Instagram has over 132 million #foodporn and over 233 million #food posts as of this writing. Add in the other social sites and blogs and there is a visual food orgy online.[18]

We all have visual hunger, a natural desire, or urge, to look at food. According to researchers Charles Spence et al., "Our brains learnt to enjoy seeing food since it would likely precede consumption. The automatic reward associated with the sight of food likely meant another day of sufficient nutrients for survival."

Food images still impact the brain. In fact, there is "a growing body of cognitive neuroscience research demonstrating the profound effect viewing such images can have on neural activity, physiological and psychological responses, and visual attention." They are finding that regular exposure to virtual food may exacerbate hunger and cause us to eat more.[19] Some experts have gone so far as to say that regular exposure to high-calorie virtual foods is contributing to the obesity epidemic.[20]

Professor Richard Magee of Sacred Heart University states that the images "draw us in because they do hit something really primal in us."[21] And the abundance of these images may be one reason women think about food more than sex. A new survey has shown that "25 percent of women think about food every half an hour, compared to the 10 percent of women who think about sex over the same time span."[22]

Interestingly, studies have also shown how thinking about food can reduce consumption and enjoyment of the same type of food. Simulating consumption can also reduce hunger.

For example, people who imagined eating a large amount of M&M's (versus a small number) significantly reduced subsequent consumption in one study.[23] And viewing 60 (versus 20) food pictures showing a specific taste experience (e.g., salty) decreased enjoyment of similar taste experiences.[24] "Similar taste" is key here. When we eat a lot of the same thing, we experience a gradual reduction in hunger, a sense of palate fatigue. In the case of the study participants, they experienced virtual palate fatigue. So, while images of food may potentially increase our hunger and our portions, perhaps they can also be used consciously to moderate our consumption.

There are also other ways to use digital technology to support our conscious choices about food. "People are pulling out their smartphones to plan meals and make healthier food choices in the moment," says Pinterest.[25] And since so many of us are using our phones in this way, many companies are taking actions to support speedy decision making. For example, Whole Foods Market has introduced a Facebook Messenger chatbot that uses artificial intelligence to converse with a robot chef to access their recipe database.[26] Want Tex-Mex ideas? Enter an emoji, and the robot will deliver suggestions in a microsecond. Now that's food for thought.

Numb and Yum: Sensory Deprivation

In modern life, our screen time has increased, and our sensory and interpersonal experiences have decreased. And we're feeling the deprivation.

Eve Turow, author of *A Taste of Generation Yum,* has a theory that in our digital-first era, many people are drawn to food as something that engages all of the senses, something tangible, and something that brings people together. With so many things out of our personal control in our lives and the abstraction of our digital habits, "food is something you can break down," she states. "You can understand it, so you can have control over the final product."[27] Turow believes this has contributed to millennials' growing obsession with food. I would argue it extends well beyond that generation.

Professor Charles Spence of Oxford University suggests that our sensory deprivation from the increase in premade and packaged food and reduction in hands-on cooking has an impact: "Might it be, then, that the current obsession with viewing others cooking on the television, and reading endless beautifully-illustrated (gastroporn) cookbooks can be framed as an implicit coping strategy designed to make up for the loss of all the cooking-related sensations (a kind of virtual comfort if you will)?"[28]

What's interesting is that the images of food we're looking at, whether in print or digital form, do not reflect our actual tables—they are an escape from what's become our real experience. Our sense of loss may very well be causing us to live vicariously through the images we're consuming. By doing so, we regain a sense of an identity we've lost touch with.

Our identities may be wrapped up with food in other ways too. There is symbolic value in many objects we buy, and there are plenty of personal or cultural meanings associated with the food we choose. It's an expression of our identity and social membership. It's a statement to ourselves as much as it is a declaration to the world.

In our worlds of plenty, we still suffer from "not enoughness." Many of us have that little voice in our head that can be highly critical, playing nasty and making us think we are inadequate. We may fill our need to be more by looking for things to make us feel better.

The grocery stores—or farmers markets or food co-ops—we shop at, food brands we buy, and even types of food we choose can be ways of expressing our identities and telling stories about ourselves. Wherever our identities are, our emotions show up alongside. Dr. Alison Armstrong, a mindfulness researcher and educator in the United Kingdom, explained to me that it's hard to separate identity from emotion. And that identity along with emotion and physical needs all influence food purchases.[29] It seems to me that given our busy schedules, identity seems to be playing into our choices more and more. I have certainly purchased the "you're a good mom" branded kids' food when I've felt guilty about working overtime.

Those purchases and shopping venues can communicate things, such as our values and what we care about, what tribe we belong to, or our social status. These items (branded grocery store shopping bags, containers of specific coffee or juice, the newest "It" vegetable) and associations (locally sourced organic ingredients, value-driven private labels) can offer social proof that we can show off or talk about even if we consume our purchases in private.

If a business or brand is in line with our current or desired identity, the purchase feels good! The symbolic value of brand association can buoy us when we feel lacking or inadequate. "We attribute symbolic value to goods; some things we buy to shore up and communicate our identity," Armstrong went on to say.

Establishing our identity through food also happens on social media, with both our authentic posts that share fun and tasty mealtime moments with our friends and with posts that are essentially self-branding performances. As the 2016 Waitrose Food and Drink Report suggests, "Food is today's hottest social currency."[30]

Toward Satisfaction

I believe that how we do one thing is how we do everything. We bring our identities, habits, preferences, and life approaches to all we do.

Our heads are full and our to-do lists long. Does this allow any room for actually tasting and enjoying what is set before us? Can we recognize our hunger even when we're not at the table? Do we understand why we are hungry and what we are really hungry for?

Learning to engage with our food in real ways along the entire path to consumption is a great place to start to deeply and authentically engage with ourselves. The food we choose, meals we create, and how and where we consume them literally become a part of us. Every day presents multiple opportunities for getting out of our heads and in touch with our senses, including our sense of self. And, starting here can influence other parts of our lives.

Paying attention and reflecting unravel confusing threads of information that have become intertwined and bring clarity about what is most important in our lives. They help us know ourselves better and identify unmet needs so we can remove the barriers to fulfilling them. That knowledge allows us to make choices (about food and beyond) that help us live with strength and vitality. It makes room for more of what makes us happy. By getting underneath the noise and noticing, we begin to understand what brings us joy. We can lighten up and laugh more and be in touch with our authentic selves as often as possible!

So, what is it you want more of? To discover that will require attention: mindfulness. Again, don't worry. Mindfulness isn't one more thing you need to add to your to-do list. It isn't about *doing*; it's about *being*. And it really is as easy as ABC! More on that next.

2

A Busy Chick's
Guide to Mindfulness

Of the tens of thousands of thoughts we have each day, the majority are not focused on the present moment. In meditation circles, the mind is referred to as a monkey mind (hopping all over), an elephant mind (strong and powerful), a puppy mind (energetic and in need of training), and the crazy roommate in our head (maybe you know her?).

Mindfulness interrupts our ongoing mental narrative to ground us in direct, sensory inputs of here and now. It allows the monkey, elephant, puppy, and roommate to be in the same room without wrecking the place.

Narrative Networks

Neuroscientists have found that we experience the world through two different neural networks.[1] We use the "narrative network" as our default approach for processing experiences through our knowledge and memory and then adding our interpretations. We use the "direct experience network" when we are attentive to and perceive inputs from our bodily sensations. Different parts of our brain become more active depending on which network we're using.

Another way of looking at the different networks is to associate the narrative network with our thinking mind and the direct experience network with our sensing mind. When we're using our thinking mind, we are thinking about ourselves, the people we know, our past and future, and how it all fits together. We may get "lost in thought." When our sensing mind is engaged, our attention goes to physical reality. We inhabit our body. In this mode, we tether our awareness to our sensory faculty, so our mind is not spinning stories.

Neither mode is better. The narrative mode helps us to set goals and plan for our futures. But we don't want to limit ourselves to only living through this approach. When we experience the moment directly through our senses, we perceive more information about the real-time events unfolding around us. Our senses are heightened and our attention increases, so the information we take in is also likely to be more accurate. We can better taste our vanilla lattes. We notice the smell of cookies in the oven turning from brilliant to burnt. We reduce our narrative meanderings (which can lead to worries and produce stress) and become present, which is calming and grounding.

Studies have shown that people who score higher on mindfulness scales have a better understanding of which mode they are using in real time and can switch between the two more easily. They also have greater cognitive control.[2] This control means they can consciously choose to take action for their long-term good rather than reacting out of habit and making short-term decisions that may not serve them later.

A lot has been written about different aspects of mindfulness over the centuries. In a world full of stimulation, it's no surprise that interest in the benefits of mindfulness has been trending upward lately.

Experts say that the surge of interest in meditation and mindfulness is the "antidote to the fast-paced tech world we live in. There's slowly been a backlash against a distracted, multi-tasking lifestyle to one that is a more self-aware, live-in-the-moment attitude."[3] Our discomfort with our distracted behavior is helping us realize we need something that serves as a counterweight, so we can find balance.

Mindfulness is a way of paying attention. It steadies us in the present by bringing our awareness to our sensory perceptions and immediate surroundings. Although its origin can be traced to the ancient Buddhist practice of meditation, these days it's often a secular practice defined by purposeful awareness—without judgment—of what's going on in the present moment.

Ellen Langer, a professor of psychology at Harvard University referred to as the "mother of mindfulness," states, "Mindfulness, as my colleagues and I study it, does not depend on meditation: it is the very simple process of noticing new things, which puts us in the present and makes us more sensitive to context and perspective. It is the essence of engagement."[4] She believes that the "illusion of certainty" is the cause of many of our problems. When we are certain and think we know everything we need, we stop paying attention. "And it's that belief that we know that keeps us from recognizing things that could work to our advantage. Everything is always changing, everything looks different from different perspectives….And once we start noticing new things, we see the things we thought we knew well, we don't really know, and then our attention naturally goes to it."[5]

Benefits of Mindfulness

- Boosts food enjoyment and mood[6]

- Helps us eat in moderation[7]

- Reduces food cravings[8]

- Helps us break bad habits[9]

- Helps us develop an awareness of hunger and fullness cues[10]

- Reduces body image concerns, emotional eating, and eating brought about by external stimuli[11]

- Supports making conscious food choices[12]

- Helps us control our responses to different emotional states[13]

- Cultivates self-acceptance[14]

- Aids in weight loss[15]

- Reduces stress[16]

- Could slow cellular aging[17]

- Significantly decreases menopausal symptoms like hot flashes[18]

Langer also reminds us that "regardless of how we get there, either through meditation or more directly by paying attention to novelty and questioning assumptions, to be mindful is to be in the present, noticing all the wonders that we didn't realize were right in front of us."[19] It's important to remember too that while meditation requires mindfulness, we can experience the benefits of mindfulness without meditating.

Unlike meditation, mindfulness doesn't require us to stop and escape to a quiet place. Mindfulness can be done anywhere, anytime, with very little time. It simply becomes part of our everyday—every *moment*—lives. By turning on our attention, we connect more deeply to the heart of each moment we are living. It's always accessible, even on the craziest days. It's as close as our next breath.

I love reading about the results researchers are finding, but I always wonder how trying to repeat their methods to achieve the results will play out for me. I wonder if maybe I'm the outlier, the girl who zigs when the majority zags. Turns out, when it comes to mindfulness, I'm part of the in crowd. My results have been like those of others.

Here are a few personal differences I've noticed since integrating mindfulness into my life:

- I have a pretty good understanding of and connection to how my body feels and reacts to different foods, levels of activity, and mental states. I can even consciously "breathe down" a stress-induced tummy ache.

- I consciously set more intentions and notice when they are in place before taking an action, like purposefully letting go of morning stress to prepare lunch with ease.

- I am more interested in eating well and eating to give my body the energy and strength it needs to live my life to the fullest, and I feel great about my food choices—even the pizza and the chocolate—because I know everything can fit in. I don't deprive myself, which is particularly important to maintaining my long-term, healthy eating habits. There is no shame, no shoulda, woulda, coulda.

- I don't automatically reject new experiences that I think will be unpleasant or cling to the familiar. I feel more adaptable and have less resistance. Life has a feeling of effortlessness.

- I've become more aware of what authentically delights, motivates, fulfills, and annoys me, and I give myself permission to create meals and other life experiences I enjoy.

My new awareness of what had been unconscious habits influencing how I chose, prepared, and consumed food prompted further investigation. With more information and better comprehension grounded in real-time observations of what was taking place within and around me, I started to make new choices, try new approaches. I dropped stale assumptions about my body and my typical diet and food lifestyle because they were outdated and no longer served me.

Before, I would eat pretty much anything I wanted. When I started to eat mindfully, I noticed that drinking milk makes me gassy and more than a serving of bread makes me tired (and gives me slow, "heavy legs" according to my tennis coach). Often my desire for a sweet after a meal is due to eating something salty, and water will satisfy me in place of something sugary. I also realized that my body is rarely hungry enough for a typical-size dinner. My tummy is often satisfied with soup, nice cheese, and a slice of baguette or a reduced-size portion of whatever food is served.

One of my goals was to understand how I felt before, during, and after eating. Tuning into my belly, even for a moment, calms and connects me to the physiological purpose of my noshing. I used to joke to myself that I was asking my tummy for feedback. So it was fascinating to learn that we also have a powerful "brain" in our digestive track!

Our belly-brain is called the enteric nervous system and is a complicated network of over 100 million neurons and neurochemicals that sense and control events in other parts of the body, including the brain. It does far more than process what we eat.[20]

In Japan, the midsection, specifically the area of the soft belly below the navel, is considered the seat of wisdom and the center of both physical and spiritual gravity: the *hara*. The Japanese speak of the hara as their center of knowing. They acknowledge the intelligence and intuition present in it, what people in other cultures may identify as gut feelings, butterflies, or a knot in the stomach.[21]

By mindfully putting our brain in our belly, we can listen to and access our gut intelligence at mealtime and throughout the day.

Tuning into what my belly was saying was one way I started understanding my hunger and fullness and cravings. We may think we are physically hungry when we are actually being triggered by something we see or smell, or perhaps we are looking for comfort or distraction. I have been dealing with the desire for distraction the entire time I've been writing this book: *This sentence is difficult to write; maybe I should just eat a cookie instead!*

Hunger is important to identify because hunger and fullness can impact planning, shopping, and meal prep in addition to what we eat. Our internal hunger cues and external environmental influences will impact our choices and experiences throughout the consumption journey.

Many of us have forgotten what true hunger feels like, which is not surprising considering how many inputs can influence it. Interestingly, experts across the fields of mindfulness, psychology, gastrophysics, and neuroscience all talk about different types of hunger or hunger channels.[22]

Visual Hunger. We all have the natural desire or urge to look at food. The beauty of the food matters, whether it's physical or virtual (e.g., food porn). We can satisfy this type of hunger by feasting our eyes on our food before digging in.

Nose Hunger. Our sense of smell is linked with taste. Hold your nose while eating something and notice how the taste changes. Satisfy this hunger by consciously taking in the aroma of food before and while eating.

Ear Hunger. The sounds of meal preparation can kick-start salivary glands. The crunchiness of a snack can impact enjoyment. To satisfy ear hunger, notice the sound of your food when chewing.

Mouth Hunger. Food can taste good! And as one craving for flavor is satisfied, our mouth hunger can perk back up if we switch to new tastes. To satisfy our mouth hunger, we can be aware of and have an open curiosity about the flavors and textures in our mouths as we bite, chew, and swallow.

Stomach Hunger. When our tummies rumbles, it could mean there's an absence of food there, but a growl can occur at any time on an empty or full stomach. The rumbling is from the muscular activity in the stomach and intestines and from gas moving around.[23] A good way to tell if you are really hungry is to drink a glass of water and wait 10–15 minutes. If you still have rumbles or can feel your tummy's emptiness, that's a good sign you are truly hungry.

Cellular Hunger. When our bodies need particular nutrients, there may be physical manifestations like a headache, fatigue, or irritability. Understanding this takes sensitivity and inner wisdom. Paying attention to body cravings and urges is a way to tune into this hunger and avoid getting *hangy* (hungry + angry).

Mind Hunger. Our minds are busy (and maybe stressed) thinking those 60,000 thoughts per day. Included in that number are thoughts about what we *should* be eating according to the latest research and repeated, mental narratives about what we *should not* be eating for whatever reason, whether real or imagined. Learning to calm our minds helps quiet the mental chatter and allows us to tune into what our bodies need and want.

Mindless Hunger. This is when we eat out of habit or are distracted and eat on autopilot: in front of a computer or phone screen, in front of the big screen at a movie, or maybe even outside at a ballpark. Paying attention to our actions in the present moment will interrupt mindless eating.

Emotional Hunger. Often, eating is linked to emotions. We may associate foods with treats from our past or think of them as offering a sense of relief from unpleasantness. We may have unmet emotional needs. At these times, many of us turn to food for comfort. Noticing which emotions we're experiencing can help us identify alternate activities if what is hungry is not our bodies but our hearts. True hunger builds slowly and can be satisfied by healthy choices like apples and carrots. If your desire for food comes on quickly and only a pint of Ben & Jerry's will do, you are likely not experiencing physiological hunger.

Being mindful at mealtimes and throughout the day is more than paying attention to the food we choose, prepare, and eat. It is learning to recognize hunger in its various forms. It is being able to eat without being impacted by external influences and noticing—and respecting—fullness. It's eating for enjoyment while nourishing our bodies.

Mindfulness creates space to connect mind and body. It's a chance to relax and reset.

Meal Feel

I really like pizza. I'm a Chicago girl! Choosing pizza from the frozen section of the supermarket is one of the best parts of my shopping trips: all the different possibilities of toppings and crusts. I love being in the kitchen when the heat of the oven touches my skin. Breathing in the aroma of melting cheese warms my heart. My tummy sings the moment I open the oven to smoothly slide out the colorful, perfectly crisped pie. I feel the expectant joy of tastiness to come. That's a happy pizza glow!

And when we order pizza in, I love carrying the warm, smooth boxes from the door to the kitchen. Extreme anticipation.

When the pizza is on the table, I look carefully at each slice, its size and the colors of its toppings, to decide which is best for me. That one with the big sausage bits, green peppers, and bubbly browned cheese.

I notice my empty belly grumbling. I want that pizza in my mouth, now! As I lift the slice, I breathe the aroma in deeply and pause a moment just before biting to admire the slice's pretty colors and crevices. *How many hands went into creating this slice of heaven?* I wonder. Too many to count. I silently appreciate them.

As I chew, I notice the heat and flavors. It's a bit too hot to taste fully right now. I'm eating it anyway, taking small bites and chewing slowly, and sipping water and wine between bites.

This dinner is fun with great Friday night conversation and a relaxed vibe. I'm aware that my tummy is still hungry, so I eat some salad. I like how the crispy, cool lettuce is a counterpoint to the warm, soft pizza.

After my second piece, I notice that I no longer have that anxious feed-me-immediately feeling. Do I want another piece? Is it worth getting up for? (We put the rest of the pizza back in the oven to keep it warm, and also so it's not in front of me, seductively advertising itself.)

I notice my inner urge to keep eating. I want to sit at the table longer to enjoy the conversation and Friday night decompression. I stay with the inner sensations of desire in my tummy and heart for a couple breaths while I listen to my son's knock-knock jokes. The sensations quiet down. They don't last forever. So, I decide to bypass another full piece to nibble on my son's extra crust and an apple slice instead. Then I'm perfectly satisfied.

This is what I think of as a happy pizza glow. It's fully appreciating and experiencing the deliciousness of the moment. It is a mindful experience at its best that didn't require extra planning, time, or energy. Now that I realize how easy it is to tap into these moments, I can re-create them with ease whether planning, shopping, cooking, or eating, and, when the moment starts to slip away, I can do a quick ABC check-in to get me back on track.

Easy as ABC: Mindfulness for Busy Chicks

Now that you're aware of many things influencing you from the outside, what mindfulness is, and some of its benefits, I want to share my technique for applying mindfulness to planning, shopping, preparing, and eating food. This technique allows me to experience that happy pizza glow often because I don't have to wait for all the conditions to magically align. Doing a mindful ABC check-in allows me to create those moments for myself.

A is for Attention

To instantly enter a state of mindfulness, I bring my attention to the present moment. I actively tune in to what's happening Now with open awareness.

I shift my focus from being *nowhere* to being *now-here*. Turning on my attention like this disrupts my normal mental chatter.

I imagine that my mind is a spotlight. Wherever it points, it shines a light on the focus of my attention. Normally, the light is a diffused glow, not always seeing what is in front of me as my thoughts skip along on various musings, memories, and future-planning topics. But focusing my attention on Now makes a bright, illuminating light that tethers my awareness to what is happening around me.

Focusing your attention may be a bit challenging at first. Research has shown that goldfish have longer attention spans than humans (9 seconds versus 8 seconds, respectively). Our increasing use of devices is likely contributing to this poor showing: the average human attention span fell from 12 seconds to 8 seconds in 2000, right around the time the mobile revolution began.[24]

So how does your attention span compare to a goldfish's?

Set your smartphone timer for 10 seconds and pay attention to your left thumb until the timer stops.

- Could you do it?

- How did it feel?

- Were you holding your breath during that time?

Given our lower-than-goldfish starting point, we have plenty of room to improve our attention. And doing so can enhance many experiences, from hobbies, to work, to relationships, to food. This silent clearing of our mind helps us respond *reflectively* rather than *reflexively* (fight or flight!) to situations we encounter throughout our day. By disrupting reflexive, habitual thoughts, we can choose a response that benefits us. We notice what's happening around us with more acuity, sensing nuance we may have glossed over when we didn't have space in our minds to perceive it, and breathe while doing it.

B is for Breath

Breathing is my favorite way into experiencing mindful moments.

After focusing my attention on Now, the next thing I do is take two or three full, deep belly breaths. I breathe in through my nose and out through my mouth. I sometimes put my hand on my belly while paying close attention to how the breath feels moving through my body.

As yoga practitioners have known for centuries, breath can act as an anchor for our attention, calm our body, and center our mind. Slow, deep breathing stimulates our parasympathetic system, the part of our nervous system that calms us down. In fact, scientists have proven that deep breathing affects much of our body, including the heart, the immune system, the brain, and digestion.[25] I always feel more relaxed after these two to three breaths.

If I am in the middle of a stressful situation, often I notice feeling very thirsty for breath. No surprise since when under duress, we may hold our breath or breathe shallowly, depriving our brain and body of necessary

Hello Breath

Taking three full breaths with complete attention is sometimes easy, sometimes not! But it's a place to start. You can do a Hello Breath anytime, anywhere to tether you to the present moment and to clear your head.

- Take one full breath with full attention breathing in through your nose and out through your mouth.

- Did you keep your focus on that single breath?

- Now, take a second full breath. Refocus if you need to.

  o This time observe the air flowing through your nostrils and how it feels. Is it cool? Warm?

  o How does your chest move? Did it expand? Did it contract?

  o Did you keep your focus totally on that breath?

- Take a third full breath. Fully feel the breath.

  o Sink into your body and release any tension.

  o How did that feel?

oxygen. If I let it, my body drinks in the air deeply and urgently.

Using breath as the object of my concentration, even for a few breaths, I become aware of my monkey mind's habit of jumping around. Sometimes it jumps around before the third breath is done! The simple discipline of bringing my attention back to the breath repeatedly brings me back to the calm richness of the present moment.

C is for Curiosity

So, we've focused our attention on Now and are breathing deeply and consciously to relax and shift our thoughts away from the everyday narrative. Next comes the fun part.

I like to get curious about what is happening Now. What is life presenting in this moment that I can perceive? As I get very interested in the goings-on around and within, I do so without evaluating or judging them as being good or bad.

I check out:

- **My body:** I consider the parts and the whole.

  o How do my feet, legs, back, torso, arms, shoulders, and neck feel?

- Do I notice any sensation or discomfort? Is my tummy hungry or full?

- I scan my body from my feet to my head, placing my focused attention into each body part. If I notice any tension in a part of my body, I relax it with a breath and let the tension go.

- **What's going on around me:** I put my senses on high alert.

  - What colors, sounds, textures, smells, and tastes do I observe?

  - Is there anything new from the last time I checked out this situation or object?

  - What can I observe that I may have overlooked in the past?

- **My thoughts and emotions:** I observe them as if from a distance.

  - What thinking-mind thoughts pop in to interrupt my engagement with my sensing mind?

  - Are they coming from my head- or heart-center?

  - Can I watch them show up in real time?

Once I note them, I put them aside and return to my senses.

Pretend you are observing as a new student of life, watching with what some call "bare attention" to notice the details but without judgment or comparison to how you think anything "should" be. Your "shoulds" create tension, dissatisfaction, and stress. Just drop them for now; you can pick them up in a bit.

Lean in to your perceptions. Get super intrigued about what is happening in this moment—it will never be repeated! What do you notice when you drop your assumptions and pay attention with your senses, rather than just observing life in a way that confirms your existing opinions? Perceive with fresh eyes and ears, like in those first days of a new school year, carefully and attentively noting all the happenings around you.

Use the immediate, direct experiences of the moment, including the movement of the breath, sensations in the body, sounds, smells, and tastes as anchors for your nonjudgmental attention. This facilitates a stabilized way of relating to your inner and outer experiences.[26]

With mindfulness, you take what you've noticed through bare attention and integrate it with existing knowledge to refine your perspective, to create clear comprehension.

You begin to find that your experiences change

depending on where you focus your attention. You become more wakeful, noticing switches between observing with your sensing mind and thinking thoughts with your narrative mind. Then you notice that your many thoughts don't last and that, as the observer of them, you can choose those that serve you best. For example, I can look at the dirty dishes on my counter and (a) simply notice without judgment that there are dishes there, or (b) think about my lack of time to clean up this morning and how I didn't have my act together, or (c) think about how nice it will feel when I tidy them up this evening and how lucky I am to have a quiet evening where I can relax, and maybe I'll listen to a new song that I've been enjoying while I do so.

Whatever you are focusing on is more likely to be pulled forward into the next moment.

Each moment that I compliment, that I savor, that I praise, gets me ready for another moment like that. This happier place always serves me better. I feel more at ease, make better decisions, intuit improved solutions. By practicing mindfulness, you'll eventually be able to notice your own narrative and more consciously choose your thoughts and actions, and that's what has the power to change your life.

In order to do that, I do ABC check-ins many times

throughout the day around and outside of food situations. The repetition of short moments of attentive awareness, conscious breathing, and present-minded curiosity has become habitual.

Mindfulness has helped me enjoy the moment and let it yield all its pleasures.

How Long Is an ABC?

In general, my ABC check-ins last a minute or so. Sometimes I stay with them longer, extending them through an entire activity, such as checking out at the store, cleaning the counter, or making a sandwich. When thoughts interrupt and try to pull me out of the moment (and they always do!), I note them and then consciously refocus and reinterest myself in the sensory details of here and now. All ABCs leave me feeling great: I seem to open up and lighten up; I feel calmer, more centered, and more content.

Eating can be a huge source of pleasure. As can the journey leading up to it if we allow it to be. When we are distracted and not present, we miss out on much of the sensual and emotional enjoyment that is available; aware and present, we can experience it fully. And when we open ourselves up to the fullest pleasure possible throughout our mealtime journey, we give ourselves the opportunity to create changes in our behavior that stays with us.

The next time you feel hungry, do an ABC check-in. Instead of focusing on your thumb or your breath, pay attention to your belly, specifically, your hara.

What does it say to you? And then ask, did listening to it bring you new awareness?

My hara told me that I was not really hungry at most meals. Now I can feel my hunger, and it makes my food more enjoyable.

As I asked more questions and responded to my cravings rather than reacting to them, I discovered that my cyclical desire for chocolate can be satisfied by steak, lentils, or spinach. Now I plan iron-rich meals and snacks and have dark chocolate for dessert. I also noticed that I don't benefit from the same type or quantity of food every day. My body shifts and so do my needs.

Habit

Practicing mindfulness gives me a highly attuned awareness of what kind of and how much food my body desires. But since I can't always decipher what my gall bladder is telling me and I am curious, I was very excited to find the company Habit, which provides science-based nutrition solutions based on "personal biology." I provided samples of my DNA (via saliva) and blood to their lab. In return, I got a biomarker report and personalized food guidance in an online report that analyzed my metabolism and nutritional needs. The report reinforced many choices I already make, and revealed some surprising new insights.

My hara was right in guiding me toward food like brown rice and salmon, my personalized suggestions for optimal carbs and protein. Surprisingly, they recommended more fat than I ever thought to eat, specifically increased monounsaturated fats. Luckily, I love avocados and already eat my fair share. I've also started incorporating chia seeds, one of my personal "hero foods," into puddings and cookies. They recommended I increase my fiber and eat 10 (10!) servings of non-starchy veggies per day. Hero foods that can help me meet this goal include red cabbage and snap peas—some new items to add to my meal plans.

This new data complements my mindful approach. I am starting to integrate their suggestions into meal planning while continuing to include my fave foods, and in doing so I feel like I am optimizing the nourishment I give my body and the pleasure I allow my spirit. When discussing my results with Habit's head coach and nutritionist, Jae Berman, she summarized: "True mindfulness and data are both important. They are two parts to the story. Nothing can replace genuine mindful, intuitive eating. Data can be a great part of that." Then she said what my heart was telling me: "Being tuned in through genuine mindfulness, that's the holy grail."[27]

So, when I pay attention, breathe, and get curious by asking questions that lead me to realize that I'm not actually hungry, I follow up with another question: *If I'm not hungry, what is triggering this sense of hunger, and what can I do to deal with this situation instead of eat?* Usually it's getting up from where I am and moving my body around by performing a simple task. If I am triggered by my emotions, some thoughts swirling in my head, or an environmental input, I will take an appropriate action.

I also integrate prompts, or cues, into my routine to remind me to pay attention and do an ABC check in if needed. For example, I have my phone and laptop passwords set to words that spark a sense of joy for me. I get very present when I type them. This helps me recognize my urges to check email, social sites, and so on, and see if they are distraction (time-wasting) impulses or real needs. I also use various kitchen tools as reminders to be in the moment—my mandoline slicer and wooden spoons are favorites. Slice or stir and ABC!

You can enjoy a happy pizza (or anything else) glow and access the vividness of the present at any moment if you slow your mind by doing an ABC check-in. Give it a try next time you sit down for a slice, a bowl, a glass, or a whatever. When you use this tool to create the best meal experiences, it's not just about the eating part. Consuming the food is only one part of a journey whose destination is determined by many decisions along the way.

Journaling Prompts:

1. Notice your narrative: Do an ABC check-in right now. Note when you switch from using your direct sensory experience to your narrative network. What triggered the switch? Jot down whatever narrative or urge you notice. See if you continue to recognize this trigger in future ABCs.

2. Recognize your hunger: For the next 24 hours, get present each time you think you are hungry or feel like eating. Not just at the table—anywhere you happen to be. Write down which type of hunger was driving your urge each time. Any patterns?

3. Personalize your glow: Identify a food or meal you experience with particular joy and depth. Use it to name and write down your own happy "_____" glow. This can be a touchstone for recognizing other deeply experienced mealtime moments.

3

Mindfully Managing
the Consumption Journey

We were all getting hungry. My family and friends were visiting from Chicago to join my husband and me for a week on the island of Nantucket. We rented a big, old house, and it was late afternoon. What would dinner be for our first night? We all took a deep breath of the salty sea air and decided on fresh scallops and seafood, a vegetable medley from the local farm, and whatever wine and extras we could find at the store. Out came the mobile phones for recipes and to check what fish was fresh. We would divide and conquer to gather the goods by foot, bike, and car.

I was relaxed and primed to contribute to the mission of creating dinner. At the seafood market, I smelled the deep fishiness of the day's catch. I noticed, for the first time, the vibrant brown and green shells of the sea creatures.

We compared stories when we met back at the house. Stories of bouncy cobblestones beneath bike wheels that almost tossed the wine out of the basket. Stories noting the deepening colors of rose bushes, fresh paint on fences, clouds shaped like cotton candy.

Cooking dinner was a hum of focused activity. We all had our tasks and prepared our work spaces. I felt very present when using the new-to-me knives, giving extra attention to chopping the cukes up perfectly. The kitchen seemed to come alive with happy potato scrubbing and playful banter. We all sincerely wanted to create a delicious meal for each other. Normal tense reactions to habitual annoyances didn't flare up (although the triggers were still there).

We set the dining table with blue and white place-mats and found a big candle for a centerpiece. We used the heavy silverware and left the windows open to sounds of the nearby harbor. The meal tasted better than any meal from an expensive restaurant we could have visited, and it stretched out much longer than usual as we savored the flavors we had created together. Even the semi-burnt bread was consumed with gusto, complete acceptance, and a few laughs.

Aware, present, happy.

We all remarked the next morning how even though we had had to improvise, the dinner process felt so effortless, perfect down to the details, with remarkably tasty flavors.

A couple of weeks later, my husband found Nantucket scallops at the store, and we decided to re-create the exact same meal at home. But we couldn't. The flavors were different, and we didn't enjoy it half as much. Maybe food just tastes better on vacation. But why can't we repeat this on a Tuesday night at home?

The food we put in our mouth has been on a long journey with many hands touching and influencing our experience with it before we take our first bite. The flour, salt, yeast, and other ingredients in our favorite morning bagel pass through a vast supply chain of farmers, processors, packagers, and shippers before ending up at the local bakery. The cream cheese had its own journey. That is the food's journey to consumption.

Similarly, our journey to consuming said bagel is based on many decisions and influences considered long before we take the first delicious bite. First, we start thinking about what to have for breakfast (maybe the night before), mentally going through various options, all weighted on our needs and criteria: We're out of cereal. We need extra fuel for a busy morning. Saw a yummy pic on Instagram. We decide on bagels and choose the place of purchase: *The café is a few blocks away from my regular commute. But I have a coupon code, and the store next door always has cute new shoes on display!* We choose which bagel we want from the tempting menu, when and where to eat (now or at the café? at work?), and how to prepare it (cream cheese, butter, or fresh preserves?). We even choose the environment in which we eat it: at our desk while reading emails, or maybe sitting quietly in the conference room alone for five minutes before the meeting. We choose—mindfully or not—when to stop eating: *So tasty but so filling; maybe keep some to eat with lunch.* Our food's and mind's long journeys come together at the moment of consumption. But before that moment come many others, most of which we aren't even aware.

We make over 225 food-related decisions every day about all aspects of eating.[1] There are a myriad of thoughts, emotions, and external influences surrounding these decisions, mostly happening unconsciously on mental autopilot, but happening nonetheless. The entire journey influences and impacts your result, the actual food you eat and how you enjoy it.

The four stages of the consumption journey are planning, shopping, cooking, and eating: I want to know, discover, spark ideas, and get prepared to execute. I want to shop and explore, purchase and order. I want to prepare, cook, create. And, I want to eat!

These stages likely feel familiar; we've been doing them unconsciously for many years even if we haven't been thinking about them in this framework.

Playing the Marketing Game

Did you know that big companies spend big bucks on research to deeply understand your consumption journey, so they can influence your choices and sell you their products at exactly the right moment, in the right place, with the right message? I've been in marketing a long time, and I've done this type of work for many corporations. They often really do know us better than we know ourselves.

Successful marketers are the ones who know enough about us to put the right products in front of us at the time we need them, saving us time and energy (and sometimes money). They can provide solutions to problems before those problems become big problems. But sometimes the right place, the right time, and the right message are right for them, and not necessarily right for us. So we need to be aware of what's going on around us and make our own conscious decisions.

Marketers have found that with technology, smartphones in particular, being central to our lives, our paths to decision and purchase have transformed: our journey is fragmented and nonlinear, punctuated by digital interactions and highly fluid. As discussed earlier, our digital access and habits are a huge influence in our hungry, busy lives.

While each stage of our consumption journey has always been composed of many individual moments, now many of these are definable thanks to our digital trail and clever research techniques. There are countless, fleeting, transient moments that make up the big chunks of life and which lead to, and influence, our more important, significant moments and decisions.[2] Like if we want a venti Frappuccino with whip or a tall fresh-brewed coffee with low-fat milk, arguably the most important decision of the morning.

Google has actually defined these micro-moments. They describe them as "intent-rich moments when decisions are made and preferences shaped."[3] They are "critical touch points within today's consumer journey, and when added together, they ultimately determine how that journey ends."[4] And when one journey ends, another is right behind it as we continue to refuel our bodies day after day.

Businesses' ability to identify and intervene in the micro-moments of our consumption journey underscores these moments' existence and their importance. We can give ourselves micro-moment makeovers by growing our own in-the-moment, lucid awareness of influences and impulses, in order to support our own best outcomes.

Managing Micro-Moments

Practicing mindfulness by regularly doing ABC check-ins helps us prepare for the micro-moments in our consumption journey. Being mindful at these times helps us take control of the narrative and make decisions that are in our own interest.

All the digital interruptions, marketing, and external influences may confuse and even annoy us at times, but if we consciously choose how we access and use the resulting information, it can be a valuable tool.

People are going online to raise their food IQ and find support in making better choices. There is growing digital content that encourages awareness and provides insight into how to live healthier, longer lives. The focus of people's diets is shifting to adding helpful foods rather than just eliminating foods, and digital content is supporting this evolution. For example, the numbers of searches for functional foods—foods such as turmeric, kefir, and apple cider vinegar that provide specific benefits—are on the rise.[5] Increasingly, consumers are snubbing packaged food's sugar, salt, and unpronounceable preservatives.[6] Online content has been a catalyst for this growing fixation with healthier food.[7]

I love digital media for the entertainment, education, and convenience it brings into our lives. I routinely search for recipes and meal inspiration from various sites and platforms. The abundance that it brings can be fun and helpful: delish recipes from around the globe at our fingertips, videos of celebrities cooking their vegan lunches with new superfood ingredients, access to time-saving home grocery and meal delivery. We can use it all to our benefit.

But sometimes the page-takeover ads, videos that open up and follow me while I scroll, native content that interrupts my reading, and trail-me-around-the-internet retargeting ads are more disruptive than helpful. Advertising is a fact of life; it supports free content and informs consumers about the many choices available. The potential problem is that simply being exposed to their content influences decisions, and so we must plan to be conscious buyers.

Since I have worked in advertising for many years, I know to be aware of the selling side of much of what I see. The most enlightened brands are trying to provide useful content alongside their products, a "value-based exchange" of you giving your attention to their brand in exchange for some helpful nugget of information, but everyone's priority is to sell.

We assume that we can tune out all of the approximately 360 ads we're exposed to every day, but the reality is, we note 150 of them.[8] Even when we're not paying attention to ads, they influence us. Research shows that advertisers influence our buying decisions simply by creating a good feeling about the product they want to sell to us. Ads that create positive associations, such as those in which objects or people that appeal to us surround a product, influence us to choose that product, even when we don't realize it is happening.

We choose things we feel good about. This is because life is busy, and we often do not have all the objective facts about choices. Our feelings are often a good marker of what is likely to turn out well, so if one option feels better to us, we are likely to go with it.[9] Trusting our gut is important, but it's also important to be mindful about how marketers and retailers are applying their knowledge of our neural pathways, physiology, and everyday micro-moments to influence us. Simply being aware of the selling you are seeing brings consciousness and choice: name it to tame it!

In today's overstimulated world, advertisers are using sophisticated tools that incorporate our personal data to match their message to our desires in hypertargeted ways. This can be very helpful to us: we search YouTube on our phones for "how to make green smoothies" and see mobile-friendly video ads for blenders, juice companies, or local grocery stores. Then we may see ads later in the day with coupons for those products along with links to more smoothie recipes. But this data also gives advertisers access to our mental and emotional world. They are paying for the opportunity to give us their version of what is good.

If you notice a brand mentioned within some social media or website content, look carefully to see if it is sponsored. Social media posts and articles that share entertaining or lifestyle stories that insert a brand might be paid for, even if it is not immediately clear when you read it. Think *The Truman Show*. Look at the fine print to determine if the content is actually a secret sponsorship.

When a content writer says he received any sort of compensation ($ or in-kind) for an "objective review" of a product or service, think twice about believing all of it. And even when reviewers don't note they received compensation, they may receive other perks they may not want to jeopardize by writing anything negative. This is a big deal on Amazon. They have rules to suppress pay-for-opinion reviews, but many listings are stuffed with great reviews given from folks who received discounted or free products. So look for balanced reviews and not overly rosy ones.

Look out for slanted review sites too: "Check out these honest reviews of the top 10 blenders from our expert testers!" The blog or website owners often get compensated through affiliate links or ad revenue and may give the product that provides the most revenue the best review or placement. Read with attention!

Also carefully consider whether any product will truly make you "more" or "less" of something too. "Be More" messaging is very sophisticated and taps into our desires and emotions. But sometimes a caffeinated beverage is just the sum of its ingredients—not the emotions stirred up by the ad. You are perfect just the way you are!

Your data is being collected by many of the sites, apps, and search platforms that you use and is sold, often in real time (thousandths of a second), to advertisers so that the ads you see are more and more relevant. Businesses pay a premium for the privilege of using this highly targeted data to show you personalized ads. Look for opt-out options if you prefer not to share your data.

Advertisers want to hook you. They'll buy information about you and use it to capture your attention. They would love to turn five seconds of your attention into five minutes, converting you from a mobile ad to their website or other sales platform. If what they offer is helpful, great! If it's a time sink, be conscious of it.

Beautiful food porn images are used purposefully to incite your hunger. There's nothing at all wrong with viewing these appetizing pictures, but just be conscious of their effect on your hunger: *I see therefore I eat*!

Planning for and enjoying an exquisite meal like the one we shared with loved ones in Nantucket didn't require that we throw away our cell phones and shun large food retailers; rather it was about being aware and balanced and mindful. We used the tools and resources at hand in the micro-moments of our consumption journey to create the experience *we* wanted.

Farm to Fork

So much of that day in Nantucket was about our state of being, how we approached our own consumption journey. Yet our failed attempt to re-create that experience made me freshly aware of how important another journey is—the journey of the food itself.

This is a journey I've been lucky enough to witness firsthand. I grew up in semirural Chicago exurbs, and my first job was at a local roadside farm stand. (I'm great at sorting apples and shucking corn.) Our home was surrounded by woods, fields, neighborhood horses, and cows: lots of acreage for a free-range childhood. I gathered wild strawberries and blackberries in the woods and constantly had scratches on my legs from wandering through brambles to gather them. My grandparents and parents had gardens filled with ingredients for salads, borscht, and tomato sandwiches, and my mom had sides of local beef in the deep freeze.

I'm very familiar with the smell of manure from the horses and cows next door and its use as natural fertilizer.

My husband's childhood was similar. He grew up on a hobby farm in Michigan where they didn't name the cows they would be eating for dinner, except the ones they named Hamburger (for real!). His grandparents lived in Wisconsin, also on a farm. When we were dating and visiting his grandparents, we would walk along the country road gathering wild asparagus to eat for dinner. In our youth, food was often only steps away.

Today, we find most of our food in the supermarket aisle rather than at the side of the road, and the journey it takes to reach us is longer and more complicated. Now the average grocery store produce item travels about 1,500 miles from farm to table, a long haul that uses plenty of fossil fuels and contributes to environmental pollutants.[10] The energy used in commercial food production is even greater. On top of that, production methods can strip out nutrients and flavor, and manufacturers add sugar, salt, and chemicals to add flavor back in. As more and more consumers become aware of the global food system and its environmental cost and nutritional impact on the food they eat, trends such as choosing organic, eating local, supporting sustainable farming, and understanding the ecological footprint of our habits and purchases have attracted more attention.

As mindful awareness of our consumption journey increases, we start to pay more attention to what we are eating and naturally get more curious about our food's journey: details about ingredients, origin, and production methods.

When I started paying attention, I was surprised and sad when I learned that my broccoli came all the way from China, organic cilantro paste from Australia, cornichon pickles from India, and honey from Argentina.

Mindfulness on our consumption journey leads

to thinking beyond ourselves. We start to sense how interconnected we are and how dependent we are on a planet that has limited resources. We start to note that our purchasing decisions have an impact on the environment and on lives of others. As we begin to notice and get curious about our food's journey and take in the impact, we can sort out what is important to us. We may start to think and choose differently when it comes to what we put in our carts and on our plates.

I feel lucky that I grew up so close to the sources of my food and had a hand—literally—in bringing it to my table and the tables of our friends and neighbors. Along with my growing practice of mindfulness, this formed my awareness of food's journey to my plate. Experiences like these, though, are disappearing and hard to replicate in our modern world. Now my childhood home is surrounded by suburbs, the woods and fields turned into subdivisions and shopping strips. To this day, my husband reminisces about collecting fresh, tasty raspberries for his breakfast while growing up. It sounds so esoteric and feels unattainable now.

While I may not be able to replicate those conditions, I do have the ability to maintain a conscious connection to our food through my food choices. Here are some of the approaches that work for me and my family:

- I buy local products as often as possible. I start with Massachusetts, then expand to New England, then the US, and then overseas.

- I plan menus around seasonal items.

- I organize shopping around farmers markets, local bakeries, and stores with local products whenever possible.

- I know the days of farmers markets in my area and sometimes use my smartphone to get recipe ideas when inspired by gorgeous, abundant produce that was not originally on my list.

- I sometimes get great recipe tips the closer I go to the source. Farm stands and the people who work there are great sources.

- When some food is obviously in season in Massachusetts (apple season!) and local grocery stores do not offer local items, I will walk out and shop somewhere else.

- I always look at labels to inform purchase decisions: I will only make the mistake of buying broccoli grown in China once!

- I also look for products that are grown and raised using organic, humane, and sustainable production methods.

Mindfulness helps me feel compassion for the animals, respect for our environment, and appreciation for the people involved in food production. I look for, and plan my meals and shopping around, products that also reflect my values. Prices for these products are usually higher, and so my ethics and my pocketbook often duel it out.

My decisions are contextual, and trade-offs are a part of reality. They depend on the product, menu, occasion, my schedule, and prices. Rather than buy broccoli from China, I will choose to pay a bit more for the local broccoli. If I find the price differential very high on certain items, I may change a recipe to use a smaller quantity to still go with these products.

I like learning the stories behind food brands and their journey to my plate. This helps me to understand why their prices may be higher or the product more desirable. They may tip the economic trade-off in their favor if I value their flavor, higher-quality ingredients, higher employee wages, or production methods.

There is a growing group of people who only eat foods from local sources. That's an authentic reflection of their values. I value locally sourced food items, and

I also love many foods from other places, and enjoy them with the awareness that there is a cost to bring them to my area. That's okay with me because I mindfully acknowledge both desires and find ways to balance them.

When I want flavors that only come from a specific territory in another country—like the distinctive olive oil from Puglia, Italy, or mochi rice nuggets from Japan—I make a point to appreciate the resources it takes to get it to me. I also try to find ways to blend my love of far-off foods with what's local. For example, I used to buy packaged French crepes at the grocery store. They were imported but inexpensive. Then I found a local café that makes them fresh: locally made but expensive. Now I make them at home. I dug out my recipe from a French girlfriend and found them so simple and fast to make, and so satisfying to eat thanks to the fresh eggs and milk, that I make them for breakfasts before school: locally made and cheap.

Over the years, I've learned what I need and value and how to find the foods that fit. I'm aware of the consumption journey—my own journey and the journey my food takes to reach me—and I make conscious decisions about where, when, and how I shop based on head and heart knowledge. This allows me to have my crepes and eat them too.

Journaling Prompts:

1. Note your own journey: Think about your last meal and your inner experience leading up to it. Write down all the decisions throughout the consumption journey that you remember that went into that meal: the what, when, where, how, and how much. What do you observe?

2. Focus on the food's journey: Take the same meal, and think about the food's journey. Write down where the food and its ingredients came from and the various steps it may have taken to reach you. How far and for how long has it been traveling? Does anything surprise you?

3. Evolve your journey: Where in your own consumption journey do you want to evolve? Think about this now, then come back after reading each chapter and write down mindful intentions for "be-ing" and "do-ing" in each stage:

Planning: I intend to be:

                I intend to do:

Shopping: I intend to be:

                I intend to do:

Cooking: I intend to be:

                I intend to do:

Eating: I intend to be:

                I intend to do:

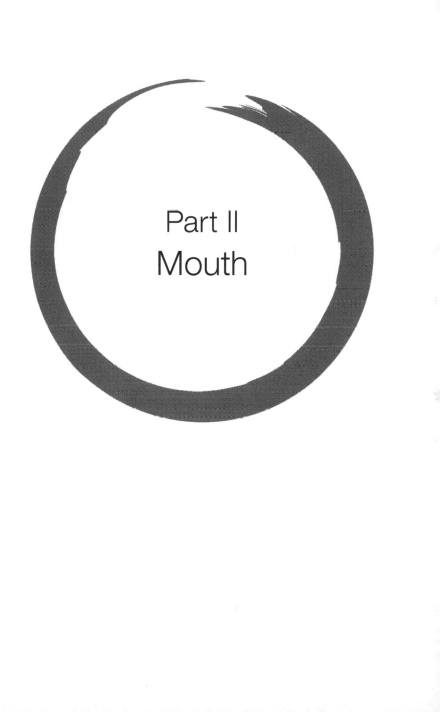

Part II
Mouth

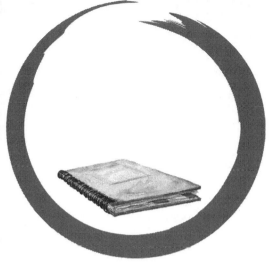

4

Mindful
Meal Planning

With our newfound mindfulness and by identifying our needs, values, expectations, and even identities, we can make decisions at key points on our consumption journey that will help us create the eating experiences we crave. Some of those key decision points involve meal planning and where to shop.

Since our shopping options affect what ingredients will be available to us, it's important to consider this first, so we know what we'll be working with in our meal planning. For example, those of us who live in large cities may have access to a wide variety of chain store retailers but little access to farmers markets. The opposite may be true for those living in rural areas. We may also choose—based on what we know about our food's journey and our values—to refrain from shopping at specific retailers or to only purchase specific types of food items (plant-based or local foods, for example). Some stores are more expensive, and some offer more bargains. Before we can plan meals, we must mindfully decide what's most important to us and which retailers are the best fit.

Whole Foods Market calls itself "America's Healthiest Grocery Store." They are the world's leader in natural and organic products with 470 stores across North America and the United Kingdom.[1] They say they are a "mission-driven company that aims to set the standards of excellence for food retailers" and that "quality is a state of mind."[2]

I have shopped at their stores for some, not all, of my groceries for over a decade. They deliver at scale the experience and feelings I had when visiting the little health food store with my mother and working at the roadside farmers market when I was in high school. Making the decision to shop at Whole Foods part of the time supports the consumption journey I wish to make. It also helps me stock my kitchen with the foods

I want to use in my meals. (Many come from the bulk bins!)

I know that I feel different when walking through Whole Foods' aisles as compared to other stores. The environment seems to make me a bit calmer, more grounded and open to investigating the many products with which I am not familiar. I prefer to shop there by myself (which is a rare luxury), so I can take my time looking around to understand their offerings and get ideas for future meal planning.

For me, Whole Foods is a good option for part of my shopping. Spend some time exploring the options in your area, if you aren't already familiar with them, and find what's the best fit for you. Once you know what foods are available, who carries them, and which shopping experiences are important to you, you can use this information in your meal planning.

Whole Foods Q&A

As I've researched, thought about, and practiced what I share in this book, I've wondered if Whole Foods thinks about supporting a mindful (less mindless) customer experience within their shopping environments.

To explore this question, I spoke with Mollie Siegler, Culinary Content Editor (and a classically trained chef) at the Whole Foods headquarters. Here are a few excerpts from my conversation:

Q: How does Whole Foods think about mindfulness? Do you incorporate any elements into your stores?
A: We consider food an opportunity to pause; this is essentially how to make it enjoyable. People can do this by committing to their own cooking and eating experience, and the journey that the food took.

We have found it is helpful when food is visually appealing, and focus on the inspirational element of food. Store layouts are designed to support customers to discover on their own, to experiment or relax into a mindful space. For example, new mochi bars allow people to enjoy in the moment.

Q: *How do you support today's busy, modern woman?*
A: Our customers are really smart and engaged. Over one million people came to our site for help with meal planning in 2016!

We want to help take the stress away from making it from scratch. Using fresh product elements in addition to packaged solutions can make something personal. Make some, buy some!

We also provide products to meet customers wherever they are—rotisserie chicken with new flavors to discover, side dishes, or premade elements so customers can make their food experience their own.[3]

These answers echo my own experience. I do enjoy their environment. I am also mindful of my budget and make meal choices consciously. Luckily their environment supports making decisions calmly, with attention.

Planning Pathways

Meal planning is mostly done in our thinking mind as opposed to the direct sensing mind we tap into during meditation and mindfulness. However, we can still choose to take a breath and engage our mind and heart completely when making meal plans.

Taking a few moments to be calm and present while meal planning allows us to get in touch with deeper desires, set intentions, and cultivate their outcome. Actions based on your mindful observations at this stage can also set up major time-saving over the days ahead.

Perhaps you have practical goals like healthier snacks, new celebration ideas, lunches that nourish body and soul, more effective fuel for workouts, and fast dinners that are satisfying for everyone and stay on budget.

Do you have any desires for your state of being? Maybe feeling more ease while shopping in crowded stores, having more patience during cooking, and experiencing deeper satisfaction while eating?

Carve out some time to sit comfortably, take a couple deep breaths, and be present to your intentions surrounding these desires. What will your meals look like? How will you feel when preparing them? What will your tummy and heart say while consuming them? Write the intentions down. By fully inhabiting each moment when you plan your meals, you are more likely to manifest what you desire, have more fun, and taste more along the way.

When you notice yourself in "what do I eat" moments, try to get really present to the contents of your head and heart. Take a full breath. Are you clear on what you are looking for? Are your body, mind, or emotions asking for something special? Notice what is showing up around you in the physical or digital world—is anything here influencing you? Try to bring a sense of equanimity, staying focused on being aware and present, to your discovery process and tune in to what you may be craving on the deepest level.

Also remember to give yourself permission to learn! It's OK not to know everything; there are abundant resources at your fingertips to uncover new ideas and information about any inquiry you might have. Last weekend I wanted to use up some pears before they rotted. After an internet search, I ended up making a zippy ginger pear soufflé for dessert.

Have you ever noticed being in the store wanting to try new foods, only to end up with the same choices in your basket? It could be the stressors in the stores making it difficult to go outside of your comfort zone and discover new things. To encourage more variety, plan some new dishes in advance and make sure you add the ingredients you'll need to your shopping list.

As you plan, ask yourself: How can I make each meal more interesting to consume? Think in terms of all the senses when planning meals. By planning the interplay of flavor and texture in meals to surprise and delight the senses, you can add variety, inject novelty, and give new twists to standard fare.

Mindful meal planning is creative. It's an act of self-exploration that connects you to your past, present, and future. And as it enables you to create your mealtimes with intention, it can provide a nourishment of its own.

As often as I can, I sit in silence while planning meals, savoring the stillness and opportunity to deeply inhabit each moment. Silence is actually all around us once we understand how to find it. It's between sounds, between breaths, between thoughts, even between the words on this page. Silence helps me connect with what I most deeply desire, and it can transform a chore into an opportunity to recharge.

Even if meal planning is starting to sound like something you could enjoy, it may seem like it takes time you don't have—but if you work 50 hours a week and sleep 8 hours a night, that still leaves 62 hours to do other things! Understanding that time is available can help us be more mindful about where it goes.

Plan for Silence

- Mute the speaker on your laptop to hush all sound notifications and video ads.

- Ask your family for some quiet time.

- Gather any meal requests in advance, and understand everyone's schedule for the week so you don't need to break out of your quietude to gather information.

- Put more space between your written words. The negative (white) space on a page makes lists easier to read and can have a calming effect when writing and reading.

Practicing mindfulness actually saves time by helping us to understand what is (and is not) important about the task at hand, prioritize accordingly, and notice where we're spending time so we can be more efficient. Have you ever watched a professional chef work? Chefs must be extremely focused. Their attention is anchored to the present, but they move quickly and can accomplish many more tasks than distracted cooks. And, they make fewer mistakes!

Moving with purpose rather than panic also helps our mental pathways stay clear, so we can accurately see what needs to get done and new options for doing it. Adam Brumberg, Deputy Director of the Food and Brand Lab at Cornell University, reminds us to "make mindful decisions upfront" and to "mindfully build your environment so you can mindlessly access it."[4] I used to make way too many last minute, time-consuming, just-ran-out-of-crucial-food shopping trips before I started practicing this wholeheartedly.

I hope considering these time-saving benefits to mindfulness makes meal planning feel more doable. If the idea seems especially daunting or if you give it a try but keep having trouble making it happen, an ABC check-in might help you figure out what's holding you back.

Resistance is an internal state of contradictory thoughts or desires. When we experience it, we often make excuses or judgments and give ourselves permission to put the job off.

There will always be things we don't really want to do, and maybe at this point meal planning is simply one of those things for you. And some level of resistance to change is natural; we all experience it, and it's OK to feel! Sit with it for a bit. Mindfully explore with a check-in to see if you can gain some insight into the cause. Is there something you can do to address it? See if you can feel the resistance in your body. Many times, we can feel it physically—in our heart, belly, clenched jaw, and other areas where we tend to hold negative emotions like fear and guilt. Try to let go and unclench.

Mindfulness helps us recognize resistance in the moment, relax rather than fight it, choose a direction to go, and take the action needed to overcome the obstacle.

We can choose to do the task with full, complete, 100-percent attention and in doing so remove our mind from the agitating resistance. Don't push the resistance away; pushing against it often activates it even more. You can acknowledge that it is there and choose to be OK with allowing it to "hang out" while you focus on the task at hand: *I don't want to peel this onion, but I am going to place that thought over on the counter while I focus on this task. I'm going to focus on how smooth the onion's skin feels, the different colors of the skin, the heaviness of the knife, the sharpness of the blade, the direction of the chopping, the size of the pieces, the smell of the juice...*

We could also choose to do the task later and move our emotions into a better place through engaging with

Meal Planning Resistance Triggers

- I'm overwhelmed and don't have time.

- It's hard. My family is picky, and we don't follow the same diet.

- I can't do it right. I always have too many left-overs that go to waste.

- I'm bored and struggle to find new ideas.

Instant Solutions

- Relax rather than fight it.

- Recalibrate with an ABC check-in.

- Focus on the task at hand.

- Or, set the task aside for a while.

something that lights us up. Then we can go back to the task in a more inspired state.

The choice is yours and can be made with a lighter heart once you are aware of the internal resistance dynamics.

The moment you become aware is the moment of choice.

Be Active in Your Energy

Spending a little time planning and prepping each week helps us minimize procrastination and allows us to be flexible when plans suddenly change. We won't be aware of those 200+ daily food decisions, so building a supportive framework through mindful observation of what we want and need can help us make better decisions faster when things happen that are beyond our control.

And, mindfulness in general can help us understand how our energy ebbs and flows on a daily, weekly, monthly, and even seasonal basis. That knowledge allows us to match our most productive times to the tasks that fit them. For example, I usually cook/prep/bake for future meals at night when my mind is tired, but I still have some energy. And remember the onion: the one where we had the option of setting it aside until we were emotionally in a better place to do the task at hand? Well, the same thing goes here. By maintaining an orderly environment and planning in advance, we have the option of going with the flow of our emotions *and* energy.

Here are a few things I do and recommend during the planning phase. Match them to when they best suit your energy level:

- Make a list of where you feel stuck when preparing meals to bring the issues to the front of your consciousness. Brainstorm ways to solve the problems.

  - I need heartier weekday breakfasts done quickly: Now I make crepe batter the night before and heat it up quickly in the morning. I also bake healthy breakfast "cookies" on Monday night after coming back from the gym.

- Keep the kitchen organized to quickly understand what is available. Rotting veggies or outdated condiments mean a lack of attention to the fridge and cupboards. Time for a kitchen detox!

- Observe when you have pockets of time to do prep and plan for it. Make a habit of "meal prep Sunday or Monday" to cut up, portion, and even create and freeze meals or parts of meals.

- Note situations when time is crunched and plan to deal with it. My sister-in-law keeps a case of water and box of granola bars in her minivan to deal with inevitable changes in her kids' schedules and their dire need for food when regular mealtimes are interrupted.

- Pay attention to your resistance. If planning for a week of meals is hard, plan a couple of days at a time or choose a meal or two (for example, all breakfasts and lunches) and go with the daily flow on the other meal(s).

- Notice what you love! Keep a list of staples you always want on hand, and add new things weekly.

- Pin the weekly meal menu to the fridge or place it somewhere handy so you (and your family) can view it and don't forget.

- Make technology work for you.

  - Save your favorite online recipes in a folder, so you don't waste time searching for them again and again.

  - Amazon's Alexa can talk you through over 60,000 recipes for those times when it would be helpful to listen to a list of ingredients and instructions before making shopping decisions.

  - Take advantage of online shopping sites that deliver to eliminate travel time to the store. They often save your shopping list from week to week to make the process highly efficient.

Planning can be good fun. This is an opportunity to let our elephant and puppy minds play together: structured and strong while playfully engaged in learning. When I think about the consumption journey (mind to mouth and farm to fork), it makes choosing and planning for meals and finding places to shop enjoyable. It helps me stay in the moment, which makes it feel like I have more time. I'm not bogged down with negative, must-do pressures and emotions. I give myself the freedom to explore and find my flow. All that helps me act out my intentions.

Do you have a goal for the week, day, or meal you're planning? Maybe greater energy, less white flour, more anti-inflammatory greens, simpler preparation, expanding your standard lunch options? Remember to put your mind in your belly and pay attention to your heart-center. Feel and visualize the tasty, healthy, satisfying outcome you want.

Find some sources you trust for ideas and dependable recipes that suit your needs. And think out of the box. I used to love the recipes in my husband's *Men's Health* magazine and would peruse it when looking for ideas for the week.

Be present to the abundance of options available and remember: keep it fun!

Scratch "from Scratch"

Being open to new options can lead to helpful discoveries.

During one cold week this past winter, I wanted to make lasagna for dinner. I always loved my mother's version and was eager to serve it to my son, as well as enjoy it myself. But as I was planning to shop, I realistically looked at our busy schedule over the next several days and knew that I wouldn't have time to make it. So I bought a frozen one from Stouffer's. It was the first time I'd ever bought this product, and although the packaging was appealing and the ingredients looked wholesome, I didn't know what to expect.

I was impressed. By the taste, quality, and fact that my son gobbled it up. But I still felt a bit of "made in a factory" guilt serving it: until, that is, I spoke with Chavanne Hanson, Deputy Head, Global Public Affairs at Nestlé S.A. (which owns the Stouffer's brand) and a registered dietitian. She shared that the noodles are laid by hand on fresh-cooked red sauce by well-trained cooks, many of them women, working in the company's "big kitchens." Then the freshly layered lasagna is quickly frozen. The freezing itself acts as a natural preservative, so they don't need to add chemical preservatives.[5]

I immediately thought of when my grandmother would send fresh food home with my mother on a weekend to be frozen, so we could cook and enjoy it at the end of the week. This story about the ladies laying the noodles down one at a time (I like to imagine they are someone's mother or grandmother) and education on freezing as a preservative woke me up to the potential for goodness available even in the frozen aisle of the store.

Sometimes we are not totally aware of the full conversation in our head and heart around this issue of what we cook ourselves and what we let others cook for us. Exploring our drivers and assumptions here can be an exercise in mindfulness.

- **Are there internal or family pressures to cook meals from scratch?** Where is this coming from? What's at the bottom of it?

- **Is there resistance to choosing prepared food?** How are you defining prepared food: canned, boxed, frozen, delivered? What assumptions do you make (it's unhealthy, too expensive, not good enough)? What judgments do you make and perceive others making (it makes me look like I can't handle cooking, it's socially irresponsible, I'm fiscally irresponsible paying for someone else to make my food)?

- **Is there resistance to cooking from scratch?**
  What are the assumptions (it's too difficult, it's
  too time-consuming, I don't know how, I'm afraid
  my family won't eat it)? Do these apply to all
  types of food?

- **What are your constraints?** Time? Budget?
  Desire? Support? Are these the same every day of
  the week? Every week of the month?

Women who work are not going to quit working
outside their homes anytime soon just to free up extra
hours to cook traditional home-cooked meals. And
women who are home, whether working remotely or
taking care of their kids, have plenty of demands on
their time that often make prepared food an unavoid-
able reality. The food industry knows that we need
solutions to fit our lifestyles; we need tasty meals and
ingredients to stretch our dollar, save time, and help us
eat healthy.

Many of us want to eat food that's as fresh as possible.
"We want solutions that work for our busy lives, but not
so instant that we feel like we're phoning it in," shared
Mollie Siegler from Whole Foods.[6] While the idea of
cooking every meal from fresh, locally sourced ingredients may sound idyllic (and look lovely on Instagram
and in food magazines), this is too time-consuming for

many modern women. Unfortunately, some prepared foods can be more expensive, and some can be of questionable quality. We've got a lot of competing values and constraints going on: monkey mind is right!

Becoming aware of your assumptions and internal dialogue can help you find solutions to best suit your unique needs. There are many healthy, tasty, frozen and premade solutions available to complement fresh food. And many fresh food recipes can be created more quickly than we often realize, especially when planned ahead. Welcome what brings you peace, health, and balance and what suits your budget and time constraints.

Bring these foods into your mindful meal planning. And then get ready to go shopping!

Journaling Prompts:

1. Explore your internal assumptions: Write down three of your common behaviors that affect how you typically plan and prepare meals and the underlying assumption (e.g., I only choose prepackaged *because* I can't cook well, etc.). Are the assumptions based on up-to-date information or a sticky mental narrative? What "shoulds" and "can'ts" influence you? Pay attention to any

dissonance between head and heart for further exploration.

2. Acknowledge your external drivers: Write down three environmental influences and constraints that affect how you typically prepare food (e.g., cooked from scratch *because* that is what Dad demands, delivered *because* I don't have time for anything else, etc.). What "shoulds" and "don'ts" influence these decisions? Pay attention to any dissonance between head and heart for further exploration.

3. Plan for glow: Identify two decisions you can make in the planning phase to create more happy "____" glow next week.

4. Fill in your mindful meal planning intentions for "be-ing" and "do-ing" in the journaling prompts at the end of chapter 3.

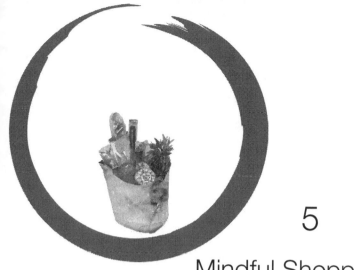

5

Mindful Shopping

When I was growing up, Thursdays were always grocery shopping days. My mother would pile us into the car with our grandparents and go through the same routine every week. We'd go to the bank, pick up her coffee at the little coffee shop, then head to Dominick's for most of the food. After a lunch stop would be Jewel for fruits and sale items, Kmart for household items, and finally the farm stand for fresh tomatoes and corn. (On top of this, trips to the health-food store and food co-op happened once a month or so.)

It took all day, my mother never rushed, and I couldn't understand why she had to go to *alllll* those stores. She said that each store was best for certain items, and every week they had different sales. She was both extremely mindful and had Old World European parents who appreciated the ritual of going to the best purveyor for the product.

My process is a bit different, a bit the same. I know which stores have the best price on fish, the freshest selection of apples, and the one that's a good choice for olive oil. I also enjoy the shopping process when I have time to do it. I like choosing the longest leeks, discovering new variations of my favorite foods, and comparing brand packaging. (My dream job would be traveling around Europe to compare yogurt aisles, testing every product and bringing the best ones home to the States where we are still behind the curve.)

But I use digital resources to supplement driving around and depend on my mobile phone for in-the-moment support. My meals are not all home-cooked, and sometimes my shopping companions are grumpier than I'm sure I ever was with my mom. While my mother seemed to naturally shop in a continual state of composure, I have had to learn to consciously create one. My shopping missions happen with less stress and more humor and grace because I've mindfully planned for them to be that way.

Captive Audience

Retail stores are all designed with a specific value system in place: theirs, not yours. When grocery shopping, we are a captive audience to the store's environment, and its design is engineered to increase sales. Research is used to determine the sights, scents, and sounds you encounter; experiences are used to trigger positive emotions: the pleasure of garden-fresh misted veggies, the fun of freshly prepared guacamole! The pioneers of merchandising found the best spots to place cameras in stores to watch customer behavior. By identifying the most viewed parts of the store, they could predict sales.[1] Do you know where your eyeballs are when you shop? Merchandisers do. And they know how to take advantage of your attention. Or inattention.

Many friends have shared how hard grocery shopping is with their kids and even their partners due to all the additional distractions: I want this! Look at this! What is this? And most of us receive near-constant dings and vibrations from our smartphone that we promptly attend to. All of this can add to the overstimulation we experience from the sights and sounds in the store, which doesn't do much for the shopping experience. But beyond that, getting interrupted while shopping actually makes us less price sensitive.[2]

Researchers have found that when we return to a product after being distracted, we have a false sense of already having thought about it and vetted it. Once we lose focus, we will often spend more on impulse purchases.[3] Said another way, stay attentive and focused to spend less on poorly considered products and impulse buys—that is, mindful behavior helps you save money!

While some interruptions are out of our control, we can still do our best to focus our attention. The best defense is a mindful offense. First, raise your awareness about what's happening.

The Path. Most of us are right-handed and naturally to want to start shopping to the right. So stores put items with sensory-stimulating bright colors or scents, like produce, flowers, and meal bars, in the front right side of the store to start us off on the route they want us to walk.[4] Buying produce first helps us feel good about making healthy decisions, so we allow ourselves more leeway for treats later in the trip. And some stores have started adding higher-priced processed items to the traditionally fresh and healthy perimeter of the store to reach us when our guard is down.[5] (Do those vegan raisin cookies really belong in the fruit section?) And, of course, the dairy is placed in the far corner to get us to walk all the way through to pick up that milk or almond milk.

Visual Cues. That perfect, ripe, banana yellow has been painstakingly researched. Customers buy the most bananas when they are Pantone color 12-0752 (Buttercup). Now banana growers plant their crops under specific conditions to produce the perfect Buttercup color."[6]

Follow the Music. Research shows that "music tempo variations can significantly affect the pace of in-store traffic flow and dollar sales volume."[7] Music can put us in a buying mood.

Follow Your Nose. The smell of freshly baking bread or roasting chickens piques hunger cues, hopefully leading to impulse purchases.[8]

Try This. The samples of food may be helping to build awareness of a specific product and slow down our shopping, but their more valuable attribute (to retailers) is stimulating our appetites.

Eye Level and Arm's Reach. Products positioned at eye level are likely to sell better, and often the more expensive options are at eye level or just below. "Eye level is buy level" is a retail mantra. Look up and down to spot deals.[9]

All the Time in the World. Have you ever noticed a lack of clocks (and windows) in some stores? The longer we stay the more we buy.[10]

It sounds basic, but don't shop hungry. Do create a shopping list. Use the list as a focal point, and remember to take some deep breaths if you start feeling overwhelmed. Bring a pen to mark off your items and reconnect to your game plan as you walk the aisles. If you didn't make a list at home, take a few minutes in the car to think through what you need and make one on your phone.

Notice your hunger level. Are you physically hungry or perhaps psychologically or emotionally hungry? Data shows that hungry grocery shoppers buy more calories, not necessarily more food. And this calorie-dense food is not usually the healthiest type.[11] Try to shop and make food decisions when you are satisfied, or acknowledge your hunger if you have it, and set a strong intention for the results that you want from your trip.

Acknowledge your soft spots and plan ahead. Are you always hungry (stressed? worn out?) at the end of the shopping trip and susceptible to the candy and drinks at checkout? Preplan to buy some fruit or other more desirable choice you can look forward to and immediately enjoy after paying.

Warning: Labels, Health Halos, and Permission to Sin

Paying mindful attention to the products you select can help you shop in line with your intention. How closely do you look at the food you place in your shopping basket? Do you ever look at the serving size and ingredients? Do you notice the promotional messages the company highlights? Do you really understand how to interpret the nutritional profile for your unique health situation?

We rely on packaging to give us helpful cues about what's inside. But marketers have engineered every detail to support sales. In fact, they are so good at it that neuroscientist Wolfram Schultz from Cambridge University suggests that junk food should be in plain packaging, because colorful packaging and attractive advertising can make sugar-rich and fatty foods irresistible to some people.[12]

But like Whole Foods, some food makers are doing more than others to educate and serve their customers.

Nestlé is the world's largest food company selling popular brands that include Stouffer's, Lean Cuisine, Gerber baby foods, Nespresso, San Pellegrino, and, of course, Nestlé Toll House chocolate morsels. The company states that they are committed to "enhancing quality of life and contributing to a healthier future."[13] I met with several employees at their headquarters in Vevey, Switzerland. They seem to have a progressively conscious approach to their business on a global scale and are evolving to address the needs of their customers who want options for convenient foods that don't sacrifice nutrition.

Nestlé was founded to help a dying child. The founder, Henri Nestlé, created a fortified infant formula, *farine lactée*, for a child who could not tolerate breast milk and was starving to death. Now, globally, they continue to focus on supporting health and wellness for individuals and families and have a corporate goal to help 50 million children lead healthier lives by 2030.[14]

By the end of 2016, they had proactively reduced sugar content by 8 percent and sodium content by 10.5 percent, and have committed to further reduce both by 5 percent and 10 percent, respectively, by 2020. This will be important as all food producers face increasing pressure from governments, health advocates, and shoppers to make products healthier.[15]

Nestlé's Maggi brand also extensively promotes home cooking and healthy meals with vegetables. The *Maggi Cooking Lesson Programme* encourages parents and kids across 35 countries to cook together with recipes and gives tips for well-balanced meals.[16] The *Maggi Diaries* is a culinary journey of Arab housewives that tells the story of how women can make a difference in people's lives through everyday cooking. By capturing the housewives' experiences through food, the video series demonstrates how every woman can be a force of change inside and outside the kitchen.

Nestlé has taken steps to educate consumers in other ways as well by creating a dedicated space, called Nestlé Nutritional Compass, on nearly all their product packages. In that space, they share insight about ingredients and tips for product enjoyment within a daily balanced diet. They also include Thoughtful Portions, a clear visual depiction of a proper portion size, and often suggest foods to complete a healthy meal. For example, their Stouffer's Family Size Lasagna with Meat and Sauce shows one-fifth of a tray as the portion size, to be accompanied by a glass of low-fat milk and green salad.

During our conversation about what Nestlé is doing to serve customers, Chavanne Hanson said, "We want to help our customers be nutritionally conscious and aware of portion sizes. For example, now we score the Nestlé Crunch chocolate bar into four 55-calorie sections. This is intended to help consumers have some now, save some for later—a more mindful approach to consumption."[17]

Some brands have taken steps that may genuinely help us consume more mindfully or consume less. And most are happy to offer smaller sizes of their products. Sometimes these sizes are convenient or meet our needs for any number of reasons, but if you're buying them with health in mind, note that smaller product sizes do not guarantee less consumption. For example, I love the cute mini-cans of sparkling wine, and friends have remarked that they think they drink less beer and soda from similarly small sizes. But researchers have found that buying multipacks of those small sizes can actually lead us to consume more.[18]

It takes attention and interest in understanding your food labels, both in store and when shopping online, to eat well and be healthy. Learning how to interpret packaging labels and identify vague and misleading information will serve you well.

Before shopping for your next meal, check out the labels of what you buy while you're still at home. See what you notice and get curious about it. Then when planning your meals and grocery list, or when you have moments of downtime (on the train, during commercial breaks, etc.), research anything you were curious about. A small investment of time up front can make your next trip easier.

Since I have a sweet tooth, I was interested to learn that a presentation at the 2014 James Beard Foundation Food Conference noted 56 different names for sugar used in ingredient lists![19] The daily allowance of sugar is not noted on ingredient lists, so we are often flying blind when analyzing a food for sugar content. And the World Health Organization is now recommending that just 5 percent or less of our total calories come from added sugar. That amounts to about 25 grams (two to three tablespoons) of sugar a day.[20] As helpful to health-conscious shoppers as product labels may be, they still aren't as helpful as they could be.

A growing trend in the industry is to provide labels that clearly and transparently state ingredients. In fact, "Clean Labeling" was Trend of the Year in 2016, according to *Food Business News*.[21] This is helpful for us, as well as companies, because there is a connection in our mind between knowing specifically what we are eating and our perception of the health and wellness benefits of the product. Clean label equals clean food, we think.

But many labels can still be misleading when they

Sugar High

A selection of the 56 different names for sugar!

- Agave

- Barley malt

- Cane juice crystals

- Corn syrup

- Dextrose

- Evaporated cane juice

- Fructose

- Galactose

- Glucose

- Honey

- Lactose

- Maltodextrin

- Maple syrup

- Molasses

- Muscovado

- Rice syrup

- Sucrose

+ *there are 16 types of "named" sugar (e.g., cane sugar, date sugar, etc.)*

add marketing buzzwords like "natural" or claims such as "part of a nutritious breakfast" on intrinsically unhealthy food. Research has shown that consumers have a heavy association between such marketing terms and health and tend to think the products containing those words are healthier than those products without them, which is not always true.[22] Pay extra attention to descriptive terms like "artisan," "clean," "earth-friendly," "pure," and "simple" on product packages and websites. The meaning of these terms is unclear; your interpretation may be different than the brand's.

A health halo is when people believe something is healthier than it really is. The health halo effect can show up when consumers believe that meals advertised as healthier have fewer calories, and compensate by choosing higher-calorie drinks, desserts, and side dishes.[23] People also tend to feel less full and eat more after consuming a food they perceive as healthy, even if it's identical to one that is marked as unhealthy. For example, they will feel hungrier after a "healthy" cookie and go on to eat more overall.[24]

Similarly, labeling products "organic" leads consumers to believe that the products are healthier than their shelf-mates. And if you're trying to avoid pesticides and extra chemicals in your food, they are. They may even have more nutrients than their conventional counterparts.[25] But research has shown that consumers generally assume that the packages marked "organic" contain fewer calories and less fat than those without the label. And this isn't necessarily the case. Organic simply refers to how the ingredients were created, prepared, or raised.[26]

Get to know your food a little deeper than surface level and double-check your assumptions!

When we make assumptions, we form habits, and let's face it, in our busy lives, we make many choices by habit. "Women can be much more aware of habits and underlying assumptions. There is no question that food is a habit and we need more awareness of our assumptions," states Dr. Alison Armstrong.[27] For example, we may assume things about the quality of all products in our shopping carts based on our impression of the store we find them in. When we focus our attention on the moment and get curious about our choices, our assumptions fall away.

Price. Do you assume all prices in a store are high or low based on the branding of the store? Do you assume one brand is more or less expensive based on advertising or competitive claims? Do you look at unit price or price per ounce? Do you assume you need to buy 3 to get the "Sale: 3 for $x ($y each)" discount? (Btw, researchers have found that "promotions that utilized multi–unit pricing ("3 for $3"), purchase limits ("Limit 12/person") and suggestive selling ("Buy 10 for your freezer") all doubled the amount consumers purchased!)[28]

Quality. Do you judge the quality of a product by its packaging? By its ingredient list? By the opinion of a friend?

Variety. Do you think the bigger store has the bigger variety of every type of product? Are the varieties carried by a store the best options available or just the ones that retailer chooses to carry for reasons that serve them but may not serve you, their customer?

Freshness. Do you assume something is fresh if it's for sale? Are the freshest products always at the back?

Sustainability. Do you think the small brands are the most socially responsible? Are the local products always the most environmentally sound?

Healthfulness. Is the organic brand or healthy-looking label really healthier? Do you understand the nutritional label?

What are your assumptions about your regular, repeated purchases? Have you fact-checked them lately?

Assumptions aren't the only things that can keep us from the outcomes we desire. There is a psychological effect called "moral licensing" where we give ourselves the OK to do something "bad" because we've been so "good." Kind of a karmic balance. This permission-to-sin effect has shown we allow ourselves to indulge after doing something positive first. Like putting the leafy greens or quinoa in our shopping basket and then heading to the ice cream.[29] The initial healthy decision helps us feel less guilty about choosing unhealthy things later. Watch your thinking around this! If you have health goals you are aiming for, remember that your purchases are a step in moving you toward (or away from) the goal and not a statement about being bad or good. And if you really want to buy the ice cream, decide to buy it from an open state of wanting to enjoy it, not with the excuse that you just loaded up on quinoa salad.

I often shop at Market Basket, a regional grocery store known for low prices and fresh veggies. The location I go to, just outside of Boston, is the biggest supermarket in New England. It's huge, always crowded, and can feel like a scavenger hunt party with the upbeat music in the background and everyone searching for their items. It's a good experience, but for every product I need, there are tons of options. This sometimes leaves me mentally exhausted: What if I make the wrong choice?

Too much decision making can overwhelm us. Decision fatigue is when the quality of our decisions start to deteriorate and we begin to make irrational trade-offs. Have you ever felt slightly paralyzed when faced with all the choices and just gave in to what felt easiest?

Researchers have found that shoppers stopped giving full attention to their decisions around 23 minutes into a simulated shopping trip.[30] After about 40 minutes of shopping, most people stop trying to be rationally selective and instead began shopping emotionally. This is when we accumulate the 50 percent of things in our cart that we never planned to buy.[31]

And also when we opt for the easy, and perhaps more expensive, choices. Hello, rotisserie chicken! (No wonder they hide the clocks.)

The idea that goods and services hold symbolic as well as functional value has been recognized by researchers for decades. We, as consumers, use product symbolism to define ourselves in various situations. We are likely aware of how we communicate, or shore up, our identity with products like cars, purses, and shoes. But do you realize that we also attribute symbolic value during grocery shopping?

I've noticed that I choose certain kids' snacks that make me feel like a health-conscious mom (even though the snack is not necessarily a healthy one!) and certain sports drinks that make me feel tougher. Choosing Grey Poupon mustard and Perrier Sparkling Water in college used to convince me I was a sophisticated sophomore. Do you ever feel that a branded store bag, loyalty program, or specific product makes you feel better about yourself in some way?

Notice if this is happening in the background of your decision process and impacting choices. By becoming aware of these assumptions in your mind, you can double-check if they are helpful to your true intentions.

The thing to look out for here is whether we are choosing products, or companies are successfully marketing to us, based on our self-perceived deficiencies. Can they only sell their product if we feel inadequate, and we need their brand because we think and feel that we just aren't smart, loving, beautiful, skinny, or in some other way good enough?

Identify your identity, and choose to eat food, not stories.

Grounded Shopping

Your food shopping experience starts your connection to cooking and eating. How well do you know the food you are choosing? Pay attention to the smell of the fruit, the colors and textures of the vegetables, and the heaviness of the bread when making your choices. Yes, stores are busy and your phone is pinging, but take a few breaths and focus on what your senses reveal to you.

Be aware of crossing the threshold when walking into the store. How is the air and light different from outside? Notice the weight of the empty basket and the smoothness of its handle. Feel your feet walking down the aisle. Notice how it feels to stretch to reach the item on the top shelf. Read the labels and grow in awareness of the actual ingredients you will consume. Listen to the music coming through the speakers; be aware of how your body and mind react to it and what it may be being used for. Think about the journey your food took before arriving in the store. Be thankful for the true abundance we have available to us. Commit to fully showing up to experience this shopping trip to choose the food that will help sustain and nourish your body for the days ahead.

When you show up, do feelings or emotions or assumptions show up too? You don't need to judge these, but rather simply notice them and choose your next action. Do you need to read the ingredients to check on your assumptions?

Be interested in what you're experiencing. Maybe thoughts around cost, crowds, or feelings of tiredness, stress, or excitement to try something new? Get to know your mind and what's running through it. You've probably had these thoughts and feelings and reactions before.

Take a few breaths. Take a few actions that reflect your intentions. Ground yourself with an ABC check-in to stay in the moment.

You will start to see marketing tactics for what they are when you look for them with calm attention. When you enter a store, set a timer on your phone for 20 minutes and notice how you feel at that point. Starting to feel some decision fatigue? Take a breath and refocus on your list!

These days any wait is an opportunity to pull out our phones and remove ourselves from our surroundings. But we can open up to some surprises while waiting. I've learned to befriend the boredom of a wait and use it to think about topics I sometimes feel I don't have time to deal with. I've also learned to relax more during a wait and accept that my day will still turn out okay, even with the delay. After all, I am here now even with the hundreds of waits and delays I've had in the past.

So accept the wait in the cold-cut section or checkout line as a chance to breathe deeply and appreciate being present in a place of such bounty, where an amazing variety of meats is offered from all over the world and where shoppers can take home enough food to last for weeks.

Smile at the child in the cart ahead of you and appreciate his cute little face.

Notice the huge assortment of colors on packages. Listen to the background sounds of people collecting food to nourish themselves and their families. Can you hear any silence within the noise? Listen carefully.

When you feel the itch to pull out the phone, stick with the sensation for a while. Notice how it really feels. Watch it. Ride it out and notice it subside.

Sometimes when I shop from a place of attention to my actions and appreciation for everything available to me in the store, I literally feel a bubbling up of joy. It can be fun to purposefully appreciate all the people working to make my shopping possible. I give a mental high five to the workers I encounter and a silent "thank you, thank you!" to the folks behind the scenes, the thousands of hands that contributed to my food's journey. I make it a point to offer a genuine smile from the heart and kind words to whoever checks me out. I almost always notice an uptick in both my and the worker's energy and attitude and have even received extra discounts without asking!

Being present to the joy in the supermarket checkout line sends you home with more lightness, more grace, which you will likely carry back into your house or apartment along with your bags of groceries. This presence will flow into your home and serve you well as you move on to the next step of your consumption journey.

It's time to get cookin'!

Journaling Prompts:

1. Be conscious of your inner state: Next time you go shopping, jot down the top narrative thoughts and emotions that occur. Notice if they impact your purchase decisions.

2. Recognize outer influences: In that same trip, mentally note which retail marketing tactics you notice. Did any of these impact purchase decisions?

3. Be aware of giving yourself permission to sin: Can you remember any examples of your use of moral licensing from past shopping trips? Pay attention in real time on your next trip.

4. Fill in your mindful shopping intentions for "be-ing" and "do-ing" in the journaling prompts at the end of chapter 3.

6

Mindful Cooking

Anyone who's ever burned a fingertip or singed off his or her eyebrows while cooking understands the importance of mindfulness when it comes to physical safety. Mindfulness and cooking are intimately related mentally too. Practicing mindfulness in the kitchen allows us to connect with our food in many of the ways my husband and I connected with our food growing up.

Feelings aside, there are practical reasons to cook at home. Studies show that people who frequently cook meals at home eat healthier and consume fewer calories than those who cook less.[1] Simply showing up in the kitchen and giving yourself permission to take time to create a nourishing meal is the most important first step. Any meal delivery or partially made meal solution that supports our limited time can still be prepared with attention when we fully inhabit each moment. When you also purposefully bring your mind and heart to however much or little you are creating, the experience can feel like an indulgent act of self-care.

Even though mindful cooking can feel great, each meal still has a resource cost: time, money, and the emotion invested in pleasing ourselves and others. Some days the pressure to perform, meal after meal, feels like a burden. Because, let's be honest, it can be a lot of work!

During my first year at university, I had a part-time job in the kitchen of my residence hall as the lettuce chopper. I faced daily mountains of lettuce to serve 1,200 residents. Let's just say I was not always into it. But I had to keep chopping. So I made a mindfulness game out of it. Anytime I noticed a negative point of view, I would let go of it and not give it any energy. I focused on the feeling of chopping, the sensory details of the lettuce, keeping my fingers away from the blade! It got easier to observe my thoughts as though from a distance, and then the negative thoughts came back less. I stopped feeling resistance. At times, "I" stopped chopping and it was just one smooth flowing activity.

Made with Love

I have felt overwhelmed when trying to prepare fresh meals quickly for hungry eaters and hear complaints like "I don't like this!" And my situation is relatively simple since there are just three of us. Sometimes the vision of Pinterest-pretty, completely cooked from scratch, healthy meals feels idealized and unrealistic.

So what to do? This may be sounding repetitive, but I really do like to take a couple of deep breaths to get out of my agitated head and send calming oxygen to my lungs and bloodstream to deal with the real-time stress. Sometimes I take a little walk to another room to calm down. Then my approach is to let the words roll off me and not judge them or myself. I know I did the best I could (no guilt here!) and that I can't control how everyone reacts. Then I focus on enjoying my own food and say that they don't have to eat it if they choose not to. (No one has ever starved in my house.)

I've also learned to introduce new foods in small portions and alongside accepted favorites when we're all relaxed, because resistance is lower and things are more fun when stress levels are down. "Just a taste" is all I request, and that usually happens. And let me tell you, joy is creating a healthy smoothie that my son thinks is a dessert.

For picky eaters, try using descriptive and evocative food names to increase enjoyment. Researchers have found that descriptively named menu items increase food sales and improve the attitudes customers have toward both the food and the restaurant. For example, "New York Style Cheesecake with Godiva Chocolate Sauce" got a more positive reaction than "Cheesecake."[2] So get creative with your descriptions!

I love to cook with my son. When he was younger, we'd start our cooking with a bit of fun to connect with how we were feeling and to become present. I made up this approach that goes with the children's song "Head, Shoulders, Knees, and Toes" because it was easy for both of us to remember. Even when he's not helping me, I do this. I put my attention into my

- **Head.** What are my thoughts? What's going on in my head?

- **Shoulders.** How does my body feel? How do my shoulders feel and how does my body feel in general? Usually I hold stress in my shoulders and neck area from being on my laptop all day.

When I put my attention here, I consciously relax and cast aside any tension.

- **Heart.** What emotions am I experiencing?

- **Tummy.** Am I hungry or full? What type of hunger? A little, a lot?

And I usually sing the fun, little song in my head while I do it!

Food that we believe has been prepared with tender loving care tastes better, according to scientists. So yes, mom's chicken soup is truly the tastiest! Researchers have found that our experience of a bodily sensation is impacted by our perception of the person delivering it—assumed good intentions can increase pleasure, make food taste better, and also decrease pain. (For example, shots administered by sweet nurses were less painful.)[3] And the mere act of anticipating eating something tasty helps us absorb more nutrients from a meal. This is because our anticipation of delectable smells and flavors stimulates our digestive system making it more efficient at absorbing nutrients.[4] Try sharing your delicious-sounding meal plans ahead of time to kick-start the enjoyment.

And when you find that there are too many cooks in the kitchen and things start to heat up, remember that our physical experience changes depending on how we read the intent of others.[5] So calm your mind and bring your heart into your cooking. It just might soothe those savage beasts and turn complaints into compliments.

Mise en Place Your Space

A clean cooking space supports a focused cooking mind. French chefs figured this out and have codified their cooking preparation as *mise en place*—a culinary term that means "putting/setting in place." It encompasses having all ingredients measured and prepped, equipment ready and placed in a logical order, and cooking space clean and clear before beginning to cook. If you've ever watched a cooking show, you've seen this in action.

For many chefs, the phrase signifies something deeper, some even call it their religion. The focus and self-discipline of the practice helps them coordinate a tremendous number of details, often under pressure. "I know people that have it tattooed on them," says Melissa Gray, a senior at the Culinary Institute of America. "It really is a way of life ...it's a way of concentrating your mind to only focus on the aspects that you need to be working on at that moment, to kind of rid yourself of distractions."[6]

Practicing mise en place has several benefits. It supports total presence and the ability to focus on the cooking process for better, more efficient results. You can also spot missing ingredients before getting started, before it becomes too late!

Working clean is a central aspect of mise en place. That means having clean tools, a clean cutting board, and clear space before beginning to cook. Keep ingredients, such as oil, within reach and in places where you won't have to look up to grab them. Think about your flow and arrange everything accordingly. Strategically position your cookbook or iPad (with recipe page open, of course). Have your veggie-trimming bucket and trash bin handy. Look and act the part by tucking a clean towel into your apron, and clean up as you go.

Mise en placing your space has an added benefit. Studies show that we tend to eat more, and eat more indulgent foods, in cluttered, chaotic kitchens.[7] You are also more likely to eat what you see on your kitchen counter. One study found that women who had breakfast cereal sitting on their counters weighed 20 pounds more than their neighbors who didn't, and those with soft drinks sitting out weighed 24–26 pounds more! The good news? Those who had a fruit

Clean Mind, Clean Kitchen

To start making over your space, first do an ABC check-in to become present to your experience. And then, get started:

- Open the windows and breathe.

- Ditch anything that's expired (spices, canned goods, tonic water gone flat...).

- Clear out excess bags, papers, and clutter.

- Get countertops as clear as possible.

- Dust and clean, polish the silver, and add decorative elements that add joy.

- Empty fridge and cupboards. Clean thoroughly.

- Take note of food you've had for a while, and make a plan to consume it.

- Take out kitchen tools and equipment. Discard those that don't work. Give away those you don't use.

- Sharpen your knives.

- Make sure everything in and on your workspace is (a) healthful (a bowl of fruit), (b) helpful (a coffee machine used daily), or (c) joyful (flowers, a candle, a picture).

- Stay attentive and curious throughout your process.

- Notice any narratives that pop up. Put them aside for now, and enjoy the new space you are creating.

bowl weighed about 13 pounds less.[8] So declutter your kitchen and move food and drink out of sight. If you can't get rid of clutter and tidy up, put yourself consciously in control of your actions while in the room.

And watch what you eat—literally. Adding a mirror can be a way to increase mindful attention in the kitchen. When eating badly, researchers have found that the presence of a mirror induces a discomfort and lowers the perceived taste of the unhealthy food, so you may eat less.[9] I use mirrors in my kitchen as a backsplash all the way around the cooking area, in a big U shape. It brightens the room by reflecting light from the windows and happens to be positioned to also reflect my chest, tummy, and bum! With these almost always in view, I can vouch for the research results.

Interestingly, the Chinese practice of feng shui also recommends adding a mirror in the kitchen in the "command position," which enables you to see all entrances. "The use of the traditional mirror behind the stove can help with focus during cooking," feng shui expert Linda Varone told me.[10] And focus is what we want when dealing with the busyness of creating meals. Being able to see who's running in and out can be helpful too.

Surrounding ourselves with the ingredients for our meals and all those mirrors can help us stay mindful in the kitchen. That mindfulness connects us to life as it is happening, something the best cooks know intuitively and practice naturally. I've heard many cooks say they know when food is ready by "being one" with it. This knowing flows through the senses. The sound and smell of sizzling bacon, the visual browning of caramelizing onions, the feel of perfectly baked bread, and of course the many tastes.

Deeply appreciating the tangible, sensual aspect of cooking can help us shake off the fatigue of the mental marathon of the day and provide a welcome antidote

Kiss the Cook

- Take two full breaths.

- Get curious. What exactly will you be putting in your body?

- See the colors and details of the food you are handling. Have you ever looked closely at the intricate nuances of your ingredients? They can be surprisingly beautiful.

- Smell the aroma as the food is transformed by heat and blends with other ingredients.

- Listen to the sounds of the ingredients being poured, stirred, sautéed, or sizzled.

- Feel the texture, the juiciness, the heft, the softness of your ingredients as you work with them.

- Watch the colors evolve throughout the cooking process.

- Taste. Often!

- And while you're at it, when you catch a glimpse of your mindful, cooking self in one of those mirrors, blow yourself a kiss of kindness.

to flat, unblinking screen time. We can decompress and enjoy the music made by a symphony of chopping knives, opening oven doors, and boiling water. I swear my end results improve when I immerse myself in mindful full-on sensory cooking: somehow the spices have better balance, the omelette gets cooked perfectly, and the inspired secret ingredient provides the perfect finishing touch. This is all accessible through the state of open, active attention to the present moment.

When we fully engage with chopping or stirring, we can notice the raw materials we are about to eat and be more connected to the meal at the end. It can also both calm and transform our attitudes. Therapists use mindful cooking for teens to teach them to focus on something besides stressors. By giving the mind an immersive subject with plenty of sensory stimulation, our thoughts get (re)directed and our energy can lighten up.

I love my son's all-in approach to cooking. He finds utter joy in simple acts of measuring ingredients precisely, emptying them into bowls, and watching how they pour, tumble, and plop. He notices the transforming smell in the oven—"Ummm, I think the cookies are burning,"—and is always game for a highly attentive taste. While we adults tend to always see three steps ahead, taking a child-like interest and enthusiasm in the kitchen (and in other everyday actions) sparks a lot of joy and helps us be in the Now.

Creating Crave

We know we eat with our mind and senses. We can put our visual hunger to good use by creating food scenes that make healthy food more appealing. Researchers have found that exposing children to pictures of vegetables in books can have a positive impact.[11] A friend of mine in California always gave different-colored bell peppers to her son to play with, and he now loves to eat them. And creating a beautiful meal in a bowl with different colors and textures will make your own lunch feel like a photoshoot! Mindfulness is an important part of inspiration, and inspiration is what allows us to create memorable meals and the kinds of moments that both trigger memories and establish them.

When I see a beautiful lasagna, I'm reminded of my mother working in our kitchen: the sights, the smells, the tastes, the love. When my friends and I create visually appealing meals for our families, we know that today's inspiration is a gift to our children. Many years from now when my friend's son looks at a beautiful bell pepper, he won't just see it for what it is but for what it embodies.

Visual appeal can bring novelty to a meal, and as we've learned, novelty draws our attention and focus. With this in mind, I decided to change how I present food on the plate to test if I would notice the novelty and look at my food more, and if this would change my experience. I started using less expected colors for typical ingredients (like orange bell peppers), unusual ingredients as toppings (raisins on salads), and different ways of presenting food (like placing peas in their own tiny bowl on top of a plate), something cooks do in restaurants regularly but I'd never tried at home.

The result was that the unexpected elements caught my eye, and I did look more carefully. These meals got me slightly more curious and engaged in the tasting. I also felt like the food was a bit more special and that I had given myself a treat.

Because our lives are so busy and the food we eat often an afterthought, we can get used to plopping food on a plate and, screen in front of face, never give it a second look. But a mindful approach to cooking and eating encourages us to satisfy all our hungers, not just the physical one. Setting our table sets the stage for the last phase of our consumption journeys.

Food psychology and gastrophysics researchers are discovering that our dining environment can also have a dramatic influence on our consumption and experience. Here are some recommendations based on their findings combined with some of my own:

- Make the color of your tablecloth match the color of your dishes: in studies, this made people take smaller portions.[12]

- Use red to encourage portion control. People who were served food on a red plate and drinks in a red cup cut calorie consumption by 40 percent. Even having chocolate on the plate did not change results.[13]

- Eat off smallish plates. I often use salad plates rather than dinner plates to keep portions under control.

- Use lots of bowls. Eating from a bowl with a rounded bottom can make you feel full when eating less.[14] I use red aperitif bowls so we don't fill up on premeal nibbles.

- Serve most of the food from the kitchen. You will be less tempted to go for additional servings than if the food was within view.

- Eat with heavy silverware, and use a bigger fork. Foods tend to be perceived as more enjoyable when eaten with heavier utensils,[15] and also people who use bigger forks eat less.[16] I personally love the way using my heavy silver feels, and we use it for every meal.

- Use short glasses for healthy drinks like water. Use tall glasses for drinks you want to consume in more moderation. People tend to drink more from short, wide glasses as compared to tall, narrow glasses.[17] So when served at a bar, be aware of the glassware.

- Use cloth napkins. Putting a soft napkin in my lap seems to relax me, settle me in to sitting at the table.

- Enjoy a premeal ritual, such as expressing appreciation (silently or out loud). Rituals enhance our enjoyment of our food because they slightly delay our gratification, which increases our savoring.[18]

  - This also applies to posting photos of your mouth-watering meal on social media, dunking donuts in coffee, and singing before eating birthday cakes! Any action that adds a delay could be beneficial, whether or not we tend to think of it as a ritual.

Use your awareness of understanding how the mind and senses work to mindfully create personalized, crave-worthy experiences that you and your dining partners will love! It's easy when you take care in how you present the food on the plate. Start to notice how gorgeous food porn images display their ingredients (the balance of colors and textures, no slop around the edges, a few sprinkled garnishes, a nice plate, etc.), and use those tricks to make your own food more attractive. Once it's plated with attention, take a moment. Give thanks. Post a picture on social media, if that's your thing. Then stash your phone away, and eat with wholehearted attention.

Journaling Prompts:

1. Be conscious of your inner state: List three things about cooking that you do not enjoy or places where you are resistant. Next time you encounter any of them, do an ABC check-in. Record what you notice and how the experience shifts.

2. Construct a supportive environment: List two immediate ways you can make your kitchen environment more supportive of focusing fully on tasks. Does any resistance come up when thinking about this? Hang with your resistant feeling for a bit, take some deep breaths, and explore what is beneath it.

3. Create crave: List two ideas you can try this week when cooking to bring more sensorial stimulation to your plates.

4. Fill in your mindful cooking intentions for "be-ing" and "do-ing" in the journaling prompts at the end of chapter 3.

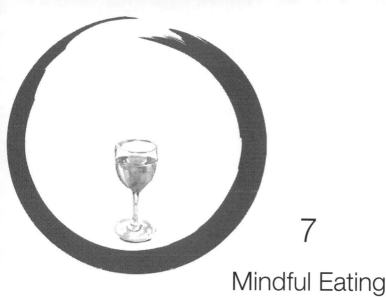

7

Mindful Eating

It's a fact: the reason we eat what we eat starts in the mind rather than the palate.[1] While our biological survival instinct still drives some food behavior, neuroscience has revealed deep crossmodal connections between the senses that are processed in the brain and impact how we perceive food experiences. Two growing fields of research, neurogastronomy and gastrophysics, underscore the importance of our minds (and mindfulness!) in what and how we eat.

Neurogastrawhatnow?

Neurogastronomy is an emerging field that merges the science and culinary worlds to examine how the brain influences our sense of taste and our eating experience. The term was created by Gordon Shepherd, a neurobiologist at Yale. His research has shown that flavor does not come only from the food and drink we put in our mouths, but also from how our minds interpret the experience. Our brains create the sensory understanding and enjoyment of what we consume. Neurogastronomists study how our brains create and distinguish flavor and how we can trick the brain to perceive food differently. This is different than the traditional approach of adding ingredients like salt, sugar, or fat to food to alter the taste.

Neurogastronomy has the potential to make healthier choices seem both tastier and more satisfying by manipulating elements like scent, temperature, and texture to fool our perception of flavor. For example, researchers in France are adding aromas to healthy food to stimulate the same reward centers in the brain as junk food—stay tuned for broccoli that tastes like a cheeseburger.[3] And chefs who apply neurogastronomy have found that ingredients can be encapsulated and distributed unevenly in a food to provide bursts of strong flavor and make your brain think the food is, for example, sweeter or saltier while using reduced quantities of sugar or salt.[4]

Gastrophysics is just as fascinating. A multidisciplinary approach, this field draws from behavioral economics, psychology, sensory science, and food science. Its name was coined by Professor Charles Spence, an experimental psychologist and head of Oxford University's Crossmodal Research Laboratory.[5]

Gastrophysics researchers are inspired by neuroscience, but are more interested in studying our real-world food behaviors in the places we are most often eating, such as restaurants and home environments. They study the impact of details relating to our dining experience beyond the food. The dining room setting, plateware, cutlery, lighting, music, even the people surrounding us all have the potential to stimulate our senses and impact us on several levels, from flavor appreciation to emotional engagement. Their research can give us a greater understanding of our relationship with food and the food choices we make on a daily basis.[6] Remember those tips in the previous chapter about setting a table top that can influence you to eat less and enjoy your meal more? We have these folks to thank for them.

The table is the end of both our mindful consumption journey and the journey of the food we consume. If we understand how our brain and body work together (or against each other), we'll enjoy this last leg of the consumption journey even more.

Got Flavor?

Taste is different than flavor, although the two words are often used interchangeably.

Taste is identified by receptors on our tongue, which distinguish between five elements: sweet, salty, bitter, sour, and umami. This tongue-centric experience is very one-dimensional. At your next meal, don't look at your food as you hold your nose and ears closed for a few chews. You may not recognize what is in your mouth based solely on taste.

Flavor is a broader experience and is constructed in our brains. It incorporates inputs from our other senses and aspects, such as memory and neurobiology, to create our rich experience of consuming food.[2]

Flavor is a powerful property that can exert control over what and how we eat. Without the contextual sensations from what we smell, see, hear, and feel, such as eating corn on the cob with our hands, to layer nuance to the input from our tongue, we don't experience our favorite foods, or any food, the same way.

Try This at Home!

More studies are showing the role of the senses in our perception of food and drink. Chivas Regal whiskey and Kitchen Theory joined the party too, investigating the many sensory inputs that impact the way drinkers perceive the flavor of whiskey, including the environment in which consumers enjoy their drink. Researchers looked at "direct" aspects, such as the color, aroma, temperature, and viscosity of the whiskey, and also at "indirect" aspects, including the glassware's shape, weight, and texture; the textures of surrounding materials (used in chairs, sofas, tablecloths, and napkins); and environmental factors of sound and lighting. These inputs all shaped the nuances of the flavor perceptions. People noticed how shifting elements made the drink taste differently.[7]

Let's revisit my Nantucket scallop meal and attempted re-creation. Professor Spence coined the term the "Provençal Rosé Paradox" based on the observation that the same wine that we consume on vacations (like the lovely rosé in Provence in Southern France) never tastes the same at home.[8] This is due to the many unique contextual stimuli we experience when on vacation, such as the different sensory environment and our state of relaxation, that just can't be repeated when we're at home. I faced the same challenge with my scallops!

Professor Spence's lab at Oxford explores how the five senses—touch, taste, smell, vision, and hearing—interact with each other. Amongst many findings, they have shown how sound is related to taste. I spoke to Janice Wang, a graduate student in Spence's lab. She shared that high-pitched sounds are associated with sweet tastes while low-pitched notes are associated with bitter. We can play those sounds to bring out the associated flavors in food because of how our senses are wired.[9]

In one study, participants tasted toffees while listening to different soundtracks. The toffees were the same, but the toffee paired with higher pitches tasted sweeter, and those eaten with lower tones tasted more bitter.[10]

In a similar study, diners eating dessert were told to dial a number to choose the flavor of their cake pops. The same cake pop tasted sweeter when dialing "1" and hearing the high-pitched tone than when dialing "2" and hearing a lower-pitched tone.[11]

This type of insight may give new utility to the smartphones sitting on our tables if we use them to summon up music to accompany and improve the taste of our meals. (My son would love any reason to add a dash of digital fun to dinner.)

This is what Spence did when he created a playlist for British Airways that was designed to enhance the flavors of the in-flight meals. Some of the pairings were based on pitch, like coffee accompanied by Plácido Domingo, since the coffee's bitterness goes well with the tenor's lower tones. He based others on the idea that the experience of eating ethnic foods is enhanced when accompanied by music from the same region. Spence says, "If you have some sort of ethnic cuisine, be it Indian, Scottish, French, Italian, then if you put people in an environment with a matching atmosphere—with French accordion music for French wine, Indian sitar music while eating Indian food—if you get the right sort of music, that will increase the perceived authenticity of the sort of food that you're eating."[12] Something we can try at home next Taco Tuesday.

Wang had many examples of how we can change our experience of a meal by changing the sounds around us. Classical music makes us experience more flavor, for example, and eating at a pub with fast music can make us drink more, faster. She emphasized the importance of noticing our environment in order to not get carried away: "At the end of the day, it comes down to mindfulness and how much attention we pay to not just the food, but our environment."[13]

Music played to create ambiance and enhance flavors

is one thing, but loud background noises suppress saltiness, sweetness, and overall enjoyment of food.[14] This was abundantly clear to me at lunch the other day when we had some very loud Kidz Bop music on for my son and his friend. My favorite sandwich from the neighboring bakery had greatly diminished flavor until we turned the music off.

While loud music may make our food less enjoyable, we may eat more when it's playing. The so-called "crunch effect" suggests that people are less likely to binge eat if they're conscious of the sound of their food. Study author Ryan Elder of Brigham Young University says, "Sound is typically labeled as the forgotten food sense, but if people are more focused on the sound the food makes, it could reduce consumption."[15]

We take in more information about our food through sound than we realize. Along with his musical experiments, Professor Spence found he could make a 15 percent difference in people's perception of a stale chip's freshness by playing them a louder crunch when they bit into it.[16] All the more reason to reduce noise and distraction and pay attention to our sensory inputs. I, for one, would like to know if it's time to throw out that bag of chips!

Researchers are also finding connections between how we feel and what we taste. We can experience the same repulsion from a rotten egg or a shameful act. According to Kendall Eskine, a cognitive psychologist at Loyola University in New Orleans, "Your brain can't tell the difference between something that tastes bad and something that makes you feel morally violated."[17] And our physical experiences can shape our perspective and judgments; for example, a yucky taste in our mouth can lead to a bad mood. Erskine continues, "I don't think we are victims to our bodies, but awareness can help us from making really harsh judgments just because we are drinking something gross."[18]

Lucky for us that data also shows that eating sweets mindfully can improve our disposition, but we'll only get the benefits if we slow down and focus on what we're doing.

Researchers have also found that eating on the go leads to weight gain. Eating while walking around triggers more overeating as compared to eating during other forms of distraction, such as watching TV or having a conversation with a friend.[19] Scientists have also found that more of the foods we eat while standing or on the go have low nutritional value and are high in empty calories.[20]

Eating is an opportunity to pause and enjoy!

Allowing ourselves to sit can feel like a small luxury with packed schedules, but it's one we should give ourselves if at all possible. Then we can concentrate on the taste sensation of each bite. We can consider and respect what we are putting in our bodies. When we sit down to eat, our stomach is in a relaxed position and our awareness is on the food, its taste, texture, and smell. This relaxation greatly improves our digestion.

But we've all experienced how illicit nibbles we eat while standing in the kitchen can be so tasty! Like those spoonfuls of peanut butter or Nutella that never make it onto bread or the cheese bits stolen from the grated pile of Gruyère. Kent Berridge, professor of biopsychology at the University of Michigan, proposes that "perhaps being out of the context of sitting down to table, lets one focus with more awareness on the sensory treat." He suggests that eating in a different environment "makes the food taste more new and vivid" and increases the pleasantness of the experience.[21] Being a daily nibbler, I have to agree. I can be completely absorbed when tasting a single spoonful of chocolate mousse while standing at the counter. I know there will only be one spoonful (for real—it's the bottom of the bowl!), and that limited quantity probably makes me extend and savor the consumption much more than when I have a bowlful for dessert. As long as we're aware of how our brain and body react under different circumstances and mindfully decide whether to belly up to the kitchen bar, all things are permissible. It is the deep attention that's most important.

The point is to limit distractions as often as possible. We have all heard this before: when you're eating turn off the TV, put away your phones, and focus on your meal. But did you realize that eating while distracted can make you take in up to 40 percent more calories than usual?[22] Also, researchers have found that if you are distracted while you eat lunch, you'll not only eat more, you will also be more likely to get hungry in the afternoon and later to eat even more at dinner.[23]

Research has shown that mindful attention helps regulate the amount of food consumed and makes it more enjoyable. Attention to what we're eating can increase eating pleasure and help us regulate the type of food and how much we eat.[24] Create a non-negotiable "food space" that is empty of distraction, a place that will allow you to fully engage and reset your mind and body.

Rest and Digest

Our best digestion occurs when the parasympathetic nervous system is active, the "rest and digest" system that helps produce a state of equilibrium in the body. This happens when we feel safe and calm. Screen-induced tension can activate the sympathetic nervous system, the fight or flight response that prepares our body for action—optimal in a true crisis but not optimal for digesting our food and absorbing the nutrients.

So, use mealtimes as opportunities to pause. Get away from the screens to lower temptation and notice the beautiful colors and the aroma of your food. Take two deep breaths and set an intention to unplug your mind-set; this alone can moderate the impact of a chaotic environment on food intake.[25] Listen to your crunching. Get interested in how the flavor changes the more you chew. Even if you choose to bring your full attention to your eating experience for only part of the meal—I work through lunch hour sometimes too— your digestive system will thank you.

Eat slowly. It can help our bodies take in more health benefits. For example, sipping tea slowly has been shown to allow the body to take in more catechins, which could help for disease prevention.[26]

Slowing down can also help moderate our consumption. Remember that it takes around 20 minutes for your body to register that you're full. Research has shown the following:

- Slow eating equals less eating. Specifically, you could save up to 70 calories by eating slowly over a half hour.[27]

- Slow eaters consume 2 ounces of food per minute, while fast eaters eat 3.1 ounces.[28]

- Fast eaters gain more weight over time than slow eaters. This may partially be because with slower eating we can better sense satisfaction.[29]

- People in one study who took 30 minutes to eat food versus 5 minutes had their rating of "fullness" rise and two gut hormones related to appetite satisfaction increased markedly.[30]

Sitting comfortably, fully tasting each bite, and giving our attention to our food and family and friends we're dining with can effortlessly slow down our intake and give our brains a chance to catch up to our bellies. It's a gift to ourselves when we step aside from the crazy pace of life to eat with attention and appreciation for the bounty on our plate and in our lives. It's not just about food. It's about drinking in and feasting on the goodness in our lives.

When we pay attention and chew our food, we get good results. Researchers have found that people who chewed their food 40 times were more satisfied after their meal as compared to those who chewed only 15 times. Those who chewed more were less hungry, less preoccupied with food, and had less desire to eat.[31] Research has also shown that increasing the number of chews before swallowing reduces meal size by up to nearly 15 percent.[32]

Not chewing and then choking was the problem that led me to write this book. After practicing lots of chewing (while sitting—most of the time at least) I can vouch that even a slight increase in the number of chews improves meal satisfaction.

Is there a way to make all this chewing less boring? A 30-second chew can certainly seem tedious. I've found that tuning into how the flavor changes can be interesting. I've noticed how some processed food has no character and dissolves quickly, with the gluten turning to sugar and my dinner tasting more like dessert. That realization has helped me switch bread preferences, and now I try to bake treats more at home because I can give them a more satisfying texture.

Chewing more also breaks down our food properly, which leads to better digestion and helps us retain more energy from the food we eat. Scientists have found that with more chews the smaller particles were more readily absorbed into the digestive system.[33]

Food may be fuel, but it's also a source of sensual and emotional pleasure. Tapping into the enjoyment of our meals through dropping distractions and paying attention to each bite pays off the crave.

Savoring things really wraps up what mindful eating is about for me. Deliberately focusing on what you're eating or drinking. Appreciating every flavor nuance. Noting each sensory detail. Slowing down to extend the pleasure of each morsel.

How can I make this bite last *foreverrr*?

Even my young son reminds me: "Savor, Mom."

Weight loss isn't the only reason to be a mindful eater, but focusing on eating pleasure can help us to consume smaller portions. The first few bites are when we enjoy our food the most. After this, each additional bite becomes less flavorful as our palate experiences "sensory adaptation"—the reduced responsiveness of our sense receptors with ongoing exposure to a stimulus. I think of it as diminishing taste returns for each bite. What's more, the final bite will determine our overall impression of a food and how much we enjoyed it.[34] So if we eat fewer bites when the flavor is more potent, we can remember the food as more enjoyable, quitting while we are ahead.

Savoring like a six-year-old also helps me recognize the importance of quality food choices. While I appreciate the convenience (and surprising quality) some packaged food can provide, I try to be discerning and gravitate toward fresh food when possible. Our palates can tell the difference between just-baked brioche from a local bakery made with fresh, minimally processed ingredients and frozen, processed brioche from a factory a thousand miles away. If you're going to extend the pleasure of your food, you may as well start with something worth savoring!

Which brings me to chocolate. Specifically, Cailler chocolate.

Cailler is Switzerland's oldest chocolate brand, and besides creating savor-worthy chocolate, they offer an interactive factory tour where visitors learn the history of milk chocolate and can do a lot of tasting. What makes the experience truly unique, though, is that they have a sensory exploration wall that explains in detail how to best appreciate consuming chocolate. Their approach is mindful to the core, and when following their tips, you can't help but more deeply enjoy and appreciate the nuance and quality of their excellent product. I'm sure this experience rings up additional sales at the store at the end of the tour.

Saaavvvvvor It!
The Cailler Chocolate Experience

Voir (look)—Notice the color, texture, designs.

Écouter (hear)—Crack off a bit and notice the sound. Different chocolates make different sounds.

Sentir (smell)—Breathe in deeply and notice the different facets of the chocolate scent.

Toucher (feel)—Notice the smoothness, hardness, weight.

Déguster (taste)—Hold the chocolate on your tongue before chewing. Breathe in through your mouth and notice the difference in taste.

Après-Goût (aftertaste)—What flavor remains?

I think people usually equate silence with boring. Yet being present enough to notice silence, even in the midst of daily sounds, can be a fascinating, powerful way to experience the world. Within silence is an interesting, absorbing stillness.

161

There is always the possibility of finding it, in the gaps between the words of your dinner companions, between the crunches of your chews, between glassware and silverware tinklings. Being aware of outer silence can quiet the noisy, inner narrative (goodbye, crazy roommate in my head). Eating in silence supports a deeper intimacy and appreciation for the food you're taking in, and I've found it develops deeper comfort with myself.

I have eaten many quiet meals. During meditation retreats, breakfasts in hotel rooms, lunches on park benches. Even while with others. When eating in silence in a group setting, I usually start out a bit self-conscious. No chitchat to break the ice. Where do I put my eyes if I'm not talking to the person across from me? I wonder if they hear my tummy grumbling. But, by the end of the meal, I have quieted my mind, fed my stomach to notable satisfaction, and feel restored and ready to return to my intense speed of work. I love this thought from Ram Dass, the author of *Be Here Now*, "The quieter you become, the more you can hear."[35]

I'm listening.

Always eating meals in silence is not the norm for me, and I don't desire to do it all the time. We have family and friends with whom to connect and share and laugh. We can still bring our attention to experience each moment the glass touches our lips to deliver a sip of water, wine, or beer, and every flavor explosion in our mouth as we eat the different food on our plate, and the feeling of a full belly laugh caused by the joke across the table. Comfy seating, dimly lit interiors, and perhaps twinkling candles draw us in to appreciate and savor the contentment of each moment, of being present with each other and ourselves.

The longest meals I've experienced have been in France. Literally hours of sitting and chatting and enjoying course after course of beautifully prepared food. These meals are full of conversation and fun, yet everyone is highly attuned to experiencing each sip and forkful. There is a lot of interest in the food and discussion about where the ingredients came from, how dishes were prepared, amusing stories about situations that arose during its preparation. All this focus on the journey of the food to the table breeds extra interest in and attention to the outcome. It also paces the meal so we have time to notice feeling full.

Cultivating mindful presence, whether while sitting in silence or laughing with friends, has the power to deepen all of our mealtime experiences.

Our consumption journey can be a full, complex

path when we become aware of the many decisions and inputs along the way. Just embrace each moment and simplify activities with ABC check-ins: Attention to the present moment, Breathing to anchor your awareness, and developing a sense of Curiosity about what you are experiencing in the Now.

Mindful eating at its best is when monkey, elephant, puppy, and crazy roommate minds sit together at the table, toast the moment, and give their compliments to the cook.

Journaling Prompts:

1. Notice your food anew: Pick one meal (like lunch or an afternoon snack) at which to do an ABC check-in for the next three days. After your check-in, continue eating mindfully with full attention on your food. Remember to use all your senses, minimize distraction, and take your time. Take notes about what comes up for you. Any trends after three days?

2. Be conscious of your inner state: Continue mindfully eating your chosen meal. Now specifically notice the narrative that shows up while eating. Write down any comments you hear without editing them. Pretend like you are taking notes on an overheard conversation with the crazy roommate in your head. What is she saying?

3. Create your environment: Write down two ways you want to try incorporating music or tableware to shift the experience of future meals.

4. Fill in your mindful eating intentions for "be-ing" and "do-ing" in the journaling prompts at the end of chapter 3.

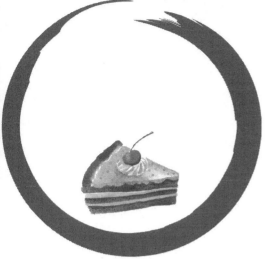

Last Bites

Making Lasting Changes

One of the biggest challenges for all of us can be making changes that stick rather than changes that fall away once a goal is reached, or after our early energy and motivation fade. With mindfulness there's no finish line to cross, no reward beyond the practice itself. As long as we want to live and eat mindfully, it will take our continued attention.

So nourish your practice.

Here are four ways you can support yourself in this ever-evolving journey:

- **Give yourself permission to reflect.** Take the time to look inward. Allowing time for reflection and meditation is not new advice, I know. Yet while we hear this often, our broader culture does not support sitting still, so it can be hard to allow yourself space to listen to your heart song. But we can create microcultures in our homes that are personalized to support self-care and nonjudgmental discovery. Carve out moments for yourself and make it a ritual. You have all the wisdom you need once you start listening.

- **Identify what you want to evolve and why it matters.** Identifying your "why" will connect you to deeply felt meaning that can carry you through. (My short-term why was to stop choking and lose some weight, and then it evolved into creating a more mindful, joyous food life for my family and me to keep us healthy.) Writing is a great practice to support deeper self-listening as you try to determine what you want to let in and what you want to release. Sometimes I use a journal. Other times I send myself daily emails that I type up in the morning before work.

- **Learn the skill of "being with" your urges.** This book has given a top-level overview on how to be with the sensations and notice the thoughts that come up around habits and cravings. For those of you who may want to explore this further and learn more about how to make lasting changes, I've included additional resources in the appendix.

- **Find your "Backyard Teacher."** Find real people who are ahead of you on the journey and who can coach you on yours. There are experts in mindfulness, mindful eating, and meditation in most of our neighborhoods as well as online. These teachers—dieticians, yoga teachers, leaders of mindfulness or meditation centers—can help you refine your practice and provide individualized support. See the appendix for additional resources.

Mindfulness is a path with no endpoint, but it can and will move us great distances. I know this because I've come a long way from choking on my way to the table.

I found it amusing when I noticed that the salmon lunch I ate today, as I finished this book, was so similar to, yet different from, the salmon lunches that initially spurred this journey. Seeing the differences reinforces that I'm succeeding in changing my approach to meals.

Before, my leftover salmon lunch was prepared in a rather messy kitchen. Its creation was uninspired: plain salmon plunked on top of a pile of lettuce. I served it on a big dinner plate; I started eating at the counter and continued eating while walking to the table; I started choking. Once I finished choking, I started working while I ate. Enjoyment level on a scale of 1–10? Maybe a 2.

Today, my leftover salmon lunch was prepared on a clear counter and made with ingredients I bought with pleasure, using a thoughtfully created plan for the week. I composed my meal with awareness and attention: salmon with dill and leeks; Swedish rye crisp with salted Irish butter; smashed potato with melted cheese; chicory and celery salad with lemon juice, olive oil, salt, and pepper; halved cherry tomatoes and raisins sprinkled in for visual fun and flavor. Finished with coffee and a chunk of chocolate. I served it on a small salad plate; I didn't start to eat until I sat down; I used heavy silverware and a cloth napkin; and I chewed consciously for most of the meal. As I ate, I looked at the food and listened to the crunches. I devoured the first bites of chocolate (yum!) and then savored the rest over several minutes with my coffee. I resumed working near the end of my meal—deadlines are approaching—but I stopped typing when I drank my coffee and nibbled my chocolate. They taste much better that way, and I like to taste. Enjoyment level on a scale of 1–10? A full-bodied 10.

Today, my lunch was filled with variety and sensory delight. This is a part of my mindful approach and of course contributed to my appreciation of the meal. But I'd venture to guess it would still be a 10, or close to it, if I instead had chosen a simple sandwich.

Mindfulness is like those higher and lower tones that reveal different flavors in the same food; it can bring our attention to the richness of what is already there. It mines the abundance of what is.

I truly hope that this book helps you bring more abundance into your life, and that it helps you on your own journey to an attentive mind, a joyous heart, and delicious meals.

Remember to just keep checking in with your Attention, Breath, and Curiosity.

Repeat.

Repeat.

Acknowledgments

A million thanks and kudos to my ace editorial team for their synergistic ability to transcend anything I could put together on my own. My deep appreciation to my editor, Cristen Iris, for her skill, commitment to excellence, and ability to put together the puzzle pieces in a masterful way. Many thanks to Robin Bethel and Kim Foster for their wordsmithing brilliance and eye for detail, and to Kiran Spees and Shiloh & team for their delightful interior designs and cover. Additional thanks to Stacy Ennis, who helped shape the initial outline and introduced me to the world of publishing.

To everyone I spoke with during official interviews and chats over coffee and wine—thank you for sharing your professional and personal insights. Kathy, Kristen, Janice, Judy, Alison, Anne, Jessica, Dao, Ellie,

Sonia, Julie, Katie, Jane, Katie, Meghan, Sarah, Jayne, Lauren, Tania—your perspectives were inspiring, thought provoking, and energizing.

Thank you to Professor Ben Brose at the University of Michigan for sharing material that expanded my understanding of the historical nuances of mindfulness.

Special thanks to Megrette Fletcher, MEd, RD, CDE, and Dr. Alison Armstrong for particularly inspiring conversations about the power of mindfulness in relation to our identities.

Thanks to my friends and family who offered wholehearted support in the midst of their busy lives.

And an extra thank you to my father, who sent pictures of best-selling books in stores and encouraged me to get my name there as well.

Heartfelt thanks to Michael for reading manuscript drafts, offering cups of tea, and picking up extra family duties so I could disappear to the library for extended writing time. And many hugs to Grayson for his enthusiastic support and frequent reminders to savor the moment.

Appendix A

More on Meditation and FAQs

I meditate 20 minutes daily to maintain my equilibrium and continue training my attention, using various breathing and concentration techniques that I learned many years ago.

For those who are interested, it can be a valuable practice. Here's a simple meditation to get you started:

- Start by sitting down somewhere quiet and comfortable.

- Keep your back straight and rest your hands on your legs. (This helps air go into your lungs with ease.)

- Gently close your eyes, and focus your internal vision on the point between your eyebrows: the point of concentration and intuition.

- Bring your attention to your breath. Notice your chest move in and out with the initial breaths. Note how the air feels in your nose—perhaps cool going in, warm going out.

- Keep your focus on each breath as you relax and breathe.

- Don't try to control it; just watch with awareness.

- You can assign a word or phrase to each inhalation and exhalation (like "in" and "out") to support your attentive watching.

- If the breath pauses naturally between inhalation and exhalation, notice the stillness.

- When your attention wanders—and it will, again and again—gently bring it back to your breath.

- This is the practice. Becoming conscious of thoughts, letting them go and refocusing your mind on the breath. Eventually, the thoughts subside and the breath slows down and you access a peaceful stillness.

- Breathe in. Breathe out. Slowly. With all your attention on your inner self.

- Try this for 30 seconds. After mastering 30

seconds, try 60. You can keep extending the time as you practice.

- Settling into a habitual 5 then 10 minutes a day is a reasonable place to start.

I've talked about the history of mindfulness and its resurgent popularity, the benefits of practicing it, and its origins in meditation, but let's pause for a moment to talk about exactly what it is and how it differs from meditation. Here are some frequently asked questions:

What is meditation? Meditation is usually associated with a sitting practice of training the mind to turn inward and focus on the present moment, often by observing the breath or repeating a word or phrase, with one-pointed focus. This quiets our thoughts and creates a still yet alert inner state. Yoga International defines it like this: "Meditation is a precise technique for resting the mind and attaining a state of consciousness that is totally different from the normal waking state…. In meditation, the mind is clear, relaxed, and inwardly focused. When you meditate, you are fully awake and alert, but your mind is not focused on the external world or on the events taking place around you."[1]

What is the difference between mindfulness and meditation? *Mindfulness* is noticing what is going on in the present moment without judging. *Meditation* is the practice of training our attention, which helps cultivate our mindfulness. I like to think of mindfulness as "eyes open" and tuning into our real-time sensory experience, while meditation is "eyes closed" and taking awareness away from our senses to a one-pointed, inward focus. There are several different types of meditation. Mindfulness is a natural by-product of a meditation practice, extending the focused awareness gained in meditation into everyday life. Meditation is not necessary for a person to be mindful, but it is helpful.

What is mindlessness? Mindlessness is not paying attention. It can also be described as when we are not engaging our mind and relying on information we've gathered in the past. We may have experienced something many times and cruise through it on mental autodrive, trusting the assumed sameness of the situation (like the commute to work). Or we may be exposed to a new situation or information and simply accept it without any thought. If we think about it (pun intended), much of how we navigate through life by the time we are adults is done in a mindless way.

What is the relaxation response? The term was created by Dr. Herbert Benson, professor, cardiologist, and founder of Harvard's Mind/Body Medical Institute. He is often credited for clearly explaining what happens in meditation and helping to bring it into the mainstream by renaming meditation the "Relaxation Response" and publishing a book of the same name. His explanation of the relaxation response is "a physical state of deep rest that changes the physical and emotional responses to stress...and [is] the opposite of the fight or flight response."[2]

Are these religious practices? For some, it is, and for others, it's not—it's more like exercise for the mind. The practice of purposefully being aware of our experience in the moment, without judgment, has been done for centuries in the East and West. While mindfulness and meditation have roots in ancient religions, they have been secularized and are now also used by athletes, performers, and people around the world who want to enjoy the benefits mentioned throughout this book.

Is this just the latest fad? Researchers are developing a greater understanding of the impact of mindfulness and meditation on the human body and the science behind it. As more data is revealed about how these practices provide repeatable, scientifically validated benefits to health and happiness, I believe they will become even more mainstream, viewed similarly to physical exercise. (Going to the gym hasn't always been as popular or accepted as it is now, either.)

Does mindfulness during mealtimes take too much time? Isn't it all about being slow and chewing forever? Mindfulness can actually help you be more productive and efficient. When you notice your actions, like chewing or chopping, you may find you want to take smaller portions or can chop more effectively.

Is it only for kale- and quinoa-eating yogis? You don't need to eat clean or live clean to enjoy the many benefits meditation and mindfulness offer. (I am no food saint!) However, as you become more aware of what you choose to buy and put in your body and how these choices make you feel during and afterward, you may start making different—healthier—choices.

Do I have to eat and do everything in silence? Not at all. Although becoming mindful may bring more peace into your life, and you may seek out more quiet moments because you like it.

Is this only for people with extreme eating issues?
Professionals successfully apply mindfulness techniques with people who have eating disorders because it has been proven to help. But anyone can apply mindfulness to evolve their relationship with themselves and the food they eat.

Will being mindful annoy my boyfriend/husband/ partner? The practice of mindfulness is invisible! No one needs to know what is happening in your mind unless you want to share it with them. The changes you experience may be so interesting, however, that you might want to talk about them.

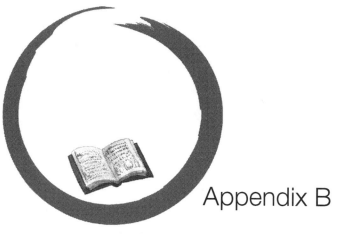

Appendix B

Additional Resources

Autobiography of a Yogi. Yogananda, Paramahansa
This is the book I read as a teenager that started my interest in and practice of meditation. It has introduced millions of readers to Eastern thought and the science of meditation. It was the one book that stayed with Steve Jobs his entire life, something he reread once a year.

Gastrophysics: The New Science of Eating. Spence, Charles. In this book, Professor Spence, an experimental psychologist at Oxford University and the inventor of gastrophysics, shares fascinating findings from his experiments to demonstrate how much the environment of our tables affects our eating experience. His work inspired part of the trajectory of this book.

Mindless Eating: Why We Eat More Than We Think and *Slim by Design: Mindless Eating Solutions for Everyday Life.* Wansink, Brian.

Professor Wansink is director of the Cornell University Food and Brand Lab. I was inspired by his surprising findings of how and why we make unconscious food decisions. Read his books to find your own inspiration—they're filled with practical ideas for supporting the behavior you intend.

The Craving Mind: From Cigarettes to Smartphones to Love—Why We Get Hooked and How We Can Break Bad Habits. Brewer, Judson.

Dr. Brewer is an acclaimed psychiatrist and neuroscientist who studied the science of addictions for 20 years. He explains in easy-to-understand and practical terms how mindfulness can interrupt addictive habits. This will change your relationship with ice cream!

The Omnivore's Dilemma: A Natural History of Four Meals. Pollan, Michael.

A thought-provoking and eye-opening look into our food's journey. His investigation of the food industry will raise your consciousness and food IQ. After reading this, you may start to imagine the taste of corn in your every bite.

The Power of Now. Tolle, Eckhart.
All of Tolle's books are written from a deep state of presence that transfers to the reader. They bring me into an actual state of experiencing what he writes about. Oprah likes him too.

Wherever You Go, There You Are: Mindfulness Meditation in Everyday Life. Kabat-Zinn, Jon.
This book was my introduction to mindfulness back in the 1990s. If you are new to mindfulness, Kabat-Zinn's multiple books provide a great introduction. He is internationally known for his work as a scientist, writer, and meditation teacher engaged in bringing mindfulness into the mainstream of medicine and society.

Eat Right Now is Dr. Judson Brewer's daily app-based program based on mindfulness and backed by science. It will help you rewire your brain to identify stress and emotional eating patterns, reduce cravings, and build sustainable, healthy habits. https://goeatrightnow.com

A Simple Way to Break a Bad Habit is a TED talk where Dr. Brewer succinctly explains how our brains form habits and how mindfulness, including the power of curiosity, can help us change behavior. https://www.youtube.com/watch?v=-moW9jvvMr4

How to Meditate on the New York Times website has clear, basic meditation instructions, follow-along audios for various meditations and mindfulness exercises, and multiple linked articles. https://www.nytimes.com/well/guides/how-to-meditate

Mindful.org and *Mindful* magazine have a rich assortment of articles and resources. They are dedicated to inspiring and guiding anyone who is interested in exploring mindfulness and applying to relationships, health and work. https://www.mindful.org/

The Center for Mindful Eating has a directory of mindful eating programs and educators. Go here to find your Backyard Teacher! http://thecenterformindfuleating.org

The Center for Mindfulness at the University of Massachusetts Medical School has online and local resources for mindfulness-based programs. http://www.umassmed.edu/cfm/

Habit will analyze your metabolic and nutrition needs via saliva and blood samples to provide a personalized biology report and nutrition plan. Getting these results was fun and highly informative; they reinforced the fit of some foods I already intuitively eat and gave me recommendations about others. I definitely recommend it! https://habit.com/

Kensho Kitchen is my company. A couple of years ago I experienced a moment of enlightenment (*kensho*, in Zen parlance) in my kitchen when a simple mandoline slicer helped me become more focused, present, and efficient while preparing dinner. This inspired me to create Kensho Kitchen, a line of products that support mindful cooking and eating. My brand is sold on Amazon, where it was awarded "Hot New Release" status, and in local boutiques. www.kenshokitchen.com

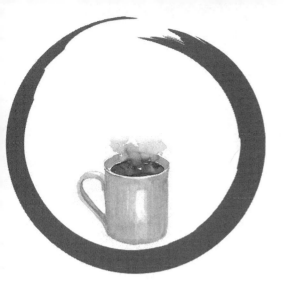

Notes

Design Note

The brushstroke circle in the design at the beginning of each chapter is an *ensō*. It is often referred to as a Zen Circle and can symbolize a variety of things. Here, it means "an expression of the moment."

Being completely present in a given moment, with the mind free from narrative thought and emotion, helps us more fully experience the richness of life. Like tasting the first bite of a juicy peach or feeling the satisfying slice of a knife through a cucumber. An ensō can also symbolize a moment when the mind is free to let the body and spirit create, such as the many opportunities for creativity along our consumption journey.

Chapter 1

1. "What's for Dinner?" Stanford University, Multidisciplinary Teaching and Research at Stanford, accessed April 14, 2014, http://news.stanford.edu/news/multi/features/food/eating.html.

2. Christine Comaford, "Got Inner Peace? 5 Ways to Get It Now," *Forbes*, April 4, 2012, https://www.forbes.com/sites/christinecomaford/2012/04/04/got-inner-peace-5-ways-to-get-it-now/#76dbc2056672.

3. Bruce Davis, "There are 50,000 Thoughts Standing Between You and Your Partner Every Day!," *HuffPost* (blog), updated July 23, 2013, http://www.huffingtonpost.com/bruce-davis-phd/healthy-relationships_b_3307916.html.

4. Brian Wansink and Jeffery Sobal, "Mindless Eating: The 200 Daily Food Decisions We Overlook," Abstract, *Environment and Behavior*, 39, no. 1 (January 2007): 106–123, https://www.researchgate.net/publication/227344004_Mindless_Eating_The_200_Daily_Food_Decisions_We_Overlook.

5. Roger Dooley, "Child Labor: Put That Baby to Work!," *Neuromarketing* (blog), *Neuroscience Marketing*, accessed September 7, 2017, https://www.neurosciencemarketing.com/blog/articles/baby-heat-maps.htm.

6. "Six Inspiring Examples of Neuromarketing Done Right," New Neuromarketing, September 6, 2016, http://www.newneuromarketing.com/six-inspiring-examples-of-neuromarketing-done-right.

7. Mark J. Perry, "Chart of the Day: Retail Sales at Grocery Stores vs. Restaurants," *AEI* (public policy

blog), March 5, 2015, https://www.aei.org/publication/
chart-day-retail-sales-grocery-stores-vs-restaurants/.

8. "Larger Portion Sizes Contribute to U.S. Obesity Problem,"
U.S. Department of Health and Human Services, National
Institutes of Health, updated February 13, 2013, https://
www.nhlbi.nih.gov/health/educational/wecan/news-events/
mattel.htm.

9. Wansink and Sobal, "Mindless Eating."

10. Allison Aubrey, "A Cluttered Kitchen Can Nudge Us to
Overeat, Study Finds," *Morning Edition,* NPR, Boise State
Public Radio, February 15, 2016, http://www.npr
.org/sections/thesalt/2016/02/15/466567647/a-cluttered
-kitchen-can-nudge-us-to-overeat-study-finds.

11. Monica Watrous, "How Boomers and Gen Z Are
Changing Food," *Food Business News,* June 30, 2016,
http://www.foodbusinessnews.net/articles/news_home/
Consumer_Trends/2016/06/How_boomers_and_Gen_Z_
are_chan.aspx?ID=%7BCE7E5EBD-336B-49A7-8FE4
-7B3D4641B1E1%7D&cck=1.

12. Margy Rochlin, "What's Up with the Cookbook Industry
These Days," *Los Angeles Times,* November 4, 2016,
http://www.latimes.com/food/dailydish/la-fo-cookbooks
-20161026-story.html.

13. B. Wansink, "Nutritional Gatekeepers and the 72%
Solution," Abstract, *Journal of the American Dietetic
Association,* 106, no. 9 (September 2006): 1324–1327,
http://www.sciencedirect.com/science/article/pii/
S0002822306017226.

14. Alexia LaFata, "Texting Has the Same Effect as an

Orgasm, That's Why You're Addicted," *Elite Daily*,
November 12, 2014, http://elitedaily.com/life/culture/
receiving-text-message-like-orgasm/845037/.

15. Pawel Piejko, "16 Mobile Market Statistics You Should
Know in 2016," Device Atlas, April 12, 2016,
https://deviceatlas.com/blog/16-mobile-market-statistics
-you-should-know-2016.

16. Alex Shellhammer, "The Need for Mobile Speed: How
Mobile Latency Impacts Publisher Revenue," Google,
"DoubleClick," September 2016, https://www.double
clickbygoogle.com/articles/mobile-speed-matters/.

17. "Jackfruit Replaces Meat, Buddha Bowls Get Big: 2017
Trends," *Progressive Grocer*, December 14, 2016,
http://www.progressivegrocer.com/research-data/research
-analysis/jackfruit-replaces-meat-buddha-bowls-get
-big-2017-trends.

18. Instagram, updated August 20, 2017, www.instagram
.com. (You must have an Instagram account to access
website.)

19. Charles Spence et al., "Eating with Our Eyes:
From Visual Hunger to Digital Satiation," *Brain and
Cognition*, 110 (December 2016): 53–63, http://www
.sciencedirect.com/science/article/pii/S0278262615300178.

20. Luke E. Stoeckel et al., "Widespread Reward-System
Activation in Obese Women in Response to Pictures of
High-Calorie Foods," Abstract, *NeuroImage*, 41, no. 2 (June
2008): 636–647, http://www.sciencedirect.com/science/
article/pii/S1053811908001638.

21. Cari Romm, "What 'Food Porn' Does to the Brain," *The*

Atlantic, April 20, 2015, https://www.theatlantic.com/health/archive/2015/04/what-food-porn-does-to-the-brain/390849/.

22. Hannamayj, "Survey: Women Think about Food More Than Sex," *Time*, December 28, 2010, http://newsfeed.time.com/2010/12/28/survey-women-think-about-food-more-than-sex/.

23. Simona Haasova et al., "Effects of Imagined Consumption and Simulated Eating Movements on Food Intake: Thoughts about Food Are Not Always of Advantage," *Frontiers in Psychology*, 7 (October 28, 2016): 1691, doi:10.3389/fpsyg.2016.01691.

24. J. Larson, J. P. Redden, and R. Elder, "Satiation from Sensory Simulation: Evaluating Foods Decreases Enjoyment of Similar Foods," *Journal of Consumer Psychology*, 24, no. 2 (2014): 188–194, https://www.researchgate.net/publication/256498174_Satiation_from_Sensory_Simulation_Evaluating_Foods_Decreases_Enjoyment_of_Similar_Foods.

25. "Jackfruit Replaces Meat."

26. John Brandon, "Whole Foods Just Launched a Messenger Chatbot for Finding Recipes with Emojis," *VentureBeat*, July 12, 2016, http://venturebeat.com/2016/07/12/whole-foods-just-launched-a-messenger-chatbot-for-finding-recipes-with-emojis/.

27. Joe Pinsker, "Why Are Millennials So Obsessed with Food?," *The Atlantic*, August 14, 2015, https://www.theatlantic.com/business/archive/2015/08/millennial-foodies/401105/.

28. Charles Spence et al., "Eating with Our Eyes."

29. Dr. Alison Armstrong (Founder and Lead Trainer, Present Minds Ltd.), in discussion with the author, January 2017.

30. "Waitrose Food and Drink Report 2016," Waitrose, accessed August 15, 2017, http://www.waitrose.com/content/dam/waitrose/Inspiration/About%20Us%20New/Waitrose%20Food%20&%20Drink%20Report.pdf.

Chapter 2

1. Norman A. S. Farb et al., "Attending to the Present: Mindfulness Meditation Reveals Distinct Neural Modes of Self-Reference," *Social Cognitive and Affective Neuroscience,* 2, no. 4 (December 1, 2007): 313–322, https://doi.org/10.1093/scan/nsm030.

2. David Rock, "The Neuroscience of Mindfulness," *Psychology Today,* October 11, 2009, https://www.psychologytoday.com/blog/your-brain-work/200910/the-neuroscience-mindfulness.

3. Kelli Kennedy, "Why Mindfulness Has Become a Trend and How You Can Do It," *Sun Sentinel,* February 26, 2016, http://www.sun-sentinel.com/health/sfl-why-mindfulness-has-become-a-trend-and-how-you-can-do-it-20160225-story.html.

4. Ellen Langer, "Mindfulness Isn't Much Harder than Mindlessness," *Harvard Business Review,* January 13, 2016, https://hbr.org/2016/01/mindfulness-isnt-much-harder-than-mindlessness.

5. Sofia Tong, "Hey Professor: Mindfulness," *The Harvard Crimson,* October 12, 2016, http://www.thecrimson.com/article/2016/10/12/hey-professor-mindfulness/.

6. "Mindful Eating of Sweets Boosts Food Enjoyment and Mood," American Mindfulness Research Association (AMRA), October 25, 2016, https://goamra.org/mindful-eating-sweets-boosts-food-enjoyment-mood/.

7. Monica Beshara, Amanda D. Hutchinson, and Carlene Wilson, "Does Mindfulness Matter? Everyday Mindfulness, Mindful Eating and Self-Reported Serving Size of Energy Dense Foods among a Sample of South Australian Adults," Abstract, *Appetite,* 67, no. 1 (August 2013): 25–29, http://www.sciencedirect.com/science/article/pii/S0195666313001207.

8. H. J. Alberts et al., "Coping with Food Cravings. Investigating the Potential of a Mindfulness-Based Intervention," Abstract, *Appetite,* 55, no. 1 (August 2010): 160–163, https://www.ncbi.nlm.nih.gov/pubmed/20493913.

9. Judson Brewer, "A Simple Way to Break a Bad Habit," University of Massachusetts Medical School Center for Mindfulness, TEDMED video, accessed February 8, 2017, http://www.umassmed.edu/cfm/a-simple-way-to-break-a-bad-habit/.

10. Kathryn M. Godfrey, Linda C. Gallo, and Niloofar Afari, "Mindfulness-Based Interventions for Binge Eating: A Systematic Review and Meta-Analysis," Abstract, *Journal of Behavioral Medicine,* 38, no. 2 (April 2015): 348–362, https://link.springer.com/article/10.1007/s10865-014-9610-5.

11. H. J. Alberts, R. Thewissen, and L. Raes, "Dealing with Problematic Eating Behaviour. The Effects of a

Mindfulness-Based Intervention on Eating Behaviour, Food Cravings, Dichotomous Thinking and Body Image Concern," Abstract, *Appetite,* 58, no. 3 (June 2012): 847–851, https://www.ncbi.nlm.nih.gov/pubmed/22265753.

12. Jean L. Kristeller and Ruth Q. Wolever, "Mindfulness-Based Eating Awareness Training for Treating Binge Eating Disorder: The Conceptual Foundation," Abstract, *Eating Disorders,* 19 (2010): 49–61, http://dx.doi.org/10.1080/10640266 .2011.533605.

13. Godfrey, Gallo, and Afari, "Mindfulness-Based Interventions."

14. Sherlyn S. Jimenez, Barbara L. Niles, and Crystal L. Park, "A Mindfulness Model of Affect Regulation and Depressive Symptoms: Positive Emotions, Mood Regulation Expectancies, and Self-Acceptance as Regulatory Mechanisms," Abstract, *Personality and Individual Differences,* 49, no. 6 (October 2010): 645–650, http://www .sciencedirect.com/science/article/pii/S0191886910002886.

15. "The 13 Best Weight-Loss Programs," *Consumer Reports,* February 2013, http://www.consumerreports.org/cro/ magazine/2013/02/lose-weight-your-way/index.htm.

16. Daphne M. Davis and Jeffrey A. Hayes, "What Are the Benefits of Mindfulness," *American Psychological Association,* 43, no. 7 (July/August 2012): 64, http://www.apa.org/ monitor/2012/07-08/ce-corner.aspx.

17. Elissa Epel et al., "Can Meditation Slow Rate of Cellular Aging? Cognitive Stress, Mindfulness, and Telomeres," *Annals of the New York Academy of Sciences,* 1172 (August 2009): 34–53, doi:10.1111/j.1749-6632.2009.04414.x.

18. James Carmody et al., "Mindfulness Training for Coping with Hot Flashes: Results of a Randomized Trial," *Menopause*, 18, no. 6 (June 2011): 611–620, https://www.ncbi.nlm.nih.gov/pmc/articles/PMC3123409/.

19. Ellen J. Langor, *Mindfulness* (Philadelphia: Da Capo Press, 2014).

20. Adam Hadhazy, "Think Twice: How the Gut's 'Second Brain' Influences Mood and Well-Being," *Scientific American*, February 12, 2010, https://www.scientificamerican.com/article/gut-second-brain/.

21. Marc David, "Are You Using the Brain in Your Belly? How Your Digestive Tract Majorly Affects Your Mood," *The Healers Journal*, June 22, 2013, http://www.thehealersjournal.com/2013/06/22/digestion-mood-brain-in-the-belly-neurotransmitters-digestive-tract/.

22. To learn more about the different types of hunger, read Jan Chozen Bays, *Mindful Eating: Rediscovering Healthy Relationships* (Boston: Shambhala Publications, 2009).

23. For more information, read Mark A. W. Andrews, "Why Does Your Stomach Growl When You Are Hungry?," *Scientific American*, https://www.scientificamerican.com/article/why-does-your-stomach-gro/.

24. Leon Watson, "Humans Have Shorter Attention Span than Goldfish, Thanks to Smartphones," *The Telegraph*, May 15, 2015, http://www.telegraph.co.uk/science/2016/03/12/humans-have-shorter-attention-span-than-goldfish-thanks-to-smart/.

25. Gretchen Cuda, "Just Breathe: Body Has a Built-In Stress Reliever," *Morning Edition*, NPR, Boise State Public Radio,

December 6, 2010, http://www.npr.org/2010/12/06/131734718/
just-breathe-body-has-a-built-in-stress-reliever.

26. New Jersey Center for Mindful Awareness, accessed April
    1, 2017, http://www.mindfulawarenessnj.com/What%20
    is%20Mindful%20Awareness%20or%20Mindfulness.html.

27. Jae Berman (Head Coach and Nutritionist, Habit), in
    discussion with the author, July 2017.

Chapter 3

1. Wansink and Sobal, "Mindless Eating."

2. Sushma Panchawati et al., "Bringing Mindfulness into
   Micro Moments," *Asia Pacific 2016—Get Connected!*,
   ESOMAR research paper, May 19, 2016. To order the report,
   visit https://2016.esomar.org/web/research_papers/
   Business-Trends_2794_Bringing-Mindfulness-into-Micro
   -Moments.php.

3. Sridhar Ramaswamy, "How Micro-Moments Are Changing
   the Rules," Google, "Think with Google," April 2015,
   https://www.thinkwithgoogle.com/marketing-resources/
   micro-moments/how-micromoments-are-changing-rules/.

4. Laura Adams, Elizabeth Burkholder, and Katie Hamilton,
   "Micro-Moments: Your Guide to Winning the Shift to
   Mobile," Google, accessed May 1, 2017, https://think.storage.
   googleapis.com/docs/micromoments-guide-to-winning
   -shift-to-mobile-download.pdf.

5. Pedro Pina, "2016 Food Trends from Google Search Data:
   The Rise of Functional Foods," Google, "Think with

Google," April 2016, https://www.thinkwithgoogle.com/consumer-insights/2016-food-trends-google/.

6.   Katherine Martinko, "Shoppers Don't Want Processed, Pre-packaged Food Anymore," TreeHugger, November 12, 2015, https://www.treehugger.com/green-food/shoppers-dont-want-processed-pre-packaged-food-anymore.html.

7.   Pina, "2016 Food Trends."

8.   Sheree Johnson, "New Research Sheds Light on Daily Ad Exposures," SJ Insights (blog), posted September 29, 2014, https://sjinsights.net/2014/09/29/new-research-sheds-light-on-daily-ad-exposures/.

9.   Art Markman, "What Does Advertising Do?," *Psychology Today*, August 31, 2010, https://www.psychologytoday.com/blog/ulterior-motives/201008/what-does-advertising-do.

10. "Boston Organics and the Local Movement," Boston Organics, accessed May 1, 2017, https://boston organics.com/how-it-works/about-local-produce.

Chapter 4

1.   "Company Info," Whole Foods Market, accessed July 1, 2017, http://www.wholefoodsmarket.com/company-info.

2.   "Declaration of Interdependence," Whole Foods Market, accessed July 1, 2017, http://www.wholefoodsmarket.com/mission-values/core-values/declaration-interdependence.

3.   Mollie Siegler (Culinary Content Editor at Whole Foods), in discussion with the author, February 2017.

4. Adam Brumberg (Deputy Director, Food and Brand Lab at Cornell University), in discussion with the author, May 2017.

5. Chavanne Hanson (Deputy Head, Global Public Affairs at Nestlé S.A.), in discussion with the author, March 2017.

6. Mollie Siegler, discussion.

Chapter 5

1. Matthew Hudson, "How to Create and Use a Retail Planogram," *The Balance*, updated July 18, 2017, https://www.thebalance.com/retail-planograms-2890336.

2. Daniella M. Kupor, Wendy Liu, and On Amir, "Risks, Interrupted," *Journal of Consumer Research*, September 3, 2013, http://dx.doi.org/10.2139/ssrn.2319465.

3. Susie Poppick, "10 Subliminal Retail Tricks You're Probably Falling For," *Money*, December 2, 2014, http://time.com/money/3069933/ways-companies-trick-you-into-buying-more/.

4. Michael Y. Park, "How to Buy Food: The Psychology of the Supermarket," *Bon Appétit*, October 30, 2014, http://www.bonappetit.com/test-kitchen/how-to/article/supermarket-psychology.

5. Carrie Dennett, "Perimeter of Grocery Stores No Longer a Safe Haven," *The Seattle Times*, September 16, 2015, http://www.seattletimes.com/life/wellness/perimeter-of-grocery-stores-no-longer-a-safe-haven/.

Notes

6. Rebecca Rupp, "Surviving the Sneaky Psychology of Supermarkets," *The Plate* (blog), *National Geographic*, June 15, 2015, http://theplate.nationalgeographic.com/2015/06/15/surviving-the-sneaky-psychology-of-supermarkets/.

7. Ronald E. Milliman, "Using Background Music to Affect the Behavior of Supermarket Shoppers," *The Journal of Marketing*, 46, no. 3 (Summer 1982): 86–91, http://freakonomics.com/media/Using%20Background%20Music%20to%20Affect%20the%20Behavior%20of%20Supermarket%20Shoppers.pdf.

8. "Can the Right Smell Lead Shoppers to Buy More Groceries?," Prolitec, December 13, 2016, https://prolitec.com/en-us/blog/can-the-right-smell-lead-shoppers-to-buy-more-groceries.

9. Gia Phua Lihua, "Eye Level Is Buy Level—The Principles of Visual Merchandising (and Shelf Placement)," *Medium*, April 3, 2016, https://medium.com/@giaphualihua/eye-level-is-buy-level-the-principles-of-visual-merchandising-and-shelf-placement-5f2fd8f7f298.

10. Rupp, "Surviving the Sneaky Psychology."

11. Aner Tal and Brian Wansink, "Fattening Fasting: Hungry Grocery Shoppers Buy More Calories, Not More Food." *JAMA International Journal of Medicine*, 173, no. 12 (2013): 1146–1148, http://jamanetwork.com/journals/jamainternalmedicine/fullarticle/1685889.

12. Ian Sample, "Sell High Calorie Foods in Plain Packaging to Beat Obesity, Says Brain Prize Winner," *The Guardian*, March 6, 2017, https://www.theguardian.com/science/2017/mar/06/obesity-sell-high-calorie

201

-foods-in-plain-packaging-says-2017-brain-prize
-winner-wolfram-schultz-peter-dayan-ray-dolan.

13. "About Us," Nestlé S.A., accessed April 28, 2017, http://
www.nestle.com/aboutus.

14. Nestlé S.A., *Nestlé in Society*, March 2017, https://
www.nestle.com/asset-library/documents/library/
documents/corporate_social_responsibility/nestle-in
-society-summary-report-2016-en.pdf.

15. Nestlé S.A., *Nestlé in Society*.

16. "Healthy Cooking, Eating and Lifestyles," Nestlé S.
A., accessed April 29, 2017, http://www.nestle.com/csv/
individuals-families/healthy-diet.

17. Chavanne Hanson, discussion.

18. Susie Poppick, "10 Subliminal Retail Tricks."

19. Robin Hilmantel, "56 Different Names for Sugar," *Women's
Health*, November 3, 2014, http://www.womens
healthmag.com/food/different-names-for-sugar.

20. World Health Organization, "WHO Calls on Countries to
Reduce Sugars Intake among Adults and Children," press
release, March 4, 2015, http://www.who.int/mediacentre/
news/releases/2015/sugar-guideline/en/.

21. Monica Watrous, "Trend of the Year: Clean Label," *Food
Business News*, accessed July 1, 2017, http://features.food
businessnews.net/corporateprofiles/2015/trend-index.html.

22. Temple Northup, "Truth, Lies, and Packaging: How Food
Marketing Creates a False Sense of Health," Abstract,
Food Studies: An Interdisciplinary Journal, 3, no. 1 (March

2014): 9–18, http://templenorthup.cgpublisher.com/product/
pub.199/prod.56.

23. Pierre Chandon and Brian Wansink, "The Biasing Health
Halos of Fast Food Restaurant Health Claims: Lower
Calorie Estimates and Higher Side–Dish Consumption
Intentions," Abstract, *Journal of Consumer Research*, 34,
no. 3 (2007): 301–314, https://foodpsychology.cornell.edu/
research/biasing-health-halos-fast%E2%80%93food
-restaurant-claims-lower-calorie-estimates-and-higher-side.

24. Jacob Suher, Raj Raghunathan, and Wayne Hoyer, "Eating
Healthy or Feeling Empty? How the 'Healthy = Less Filling'
Intuition Influences Satiety," *The Journal of the Association
for Consumer Research*, 1, no. 1 (2016), https://foodpsychology.
cornell.edu/JACR/eating_healthy_feeling_empty.

25. M. Barański et al., "Higher Antioxidant and Lower
Cadmium Concentrations and Lower Incidence of Pesticide
Residues in Organically Grown Crops: A Systematic
Literature Review and Meta-Analyses," Abstract, *The British
Journal of Nutrition*, 112, no. 5 (September 14, 2014): 794–811,
https://www.ncbi.nlm.nih.gov/pubmed/24968103.

26. Jenny Lee Wan-chen et al., "You Taste What You See: Do
Organic Labels Bias Taste Perceptions? Abstract, *Food
Quality and Preference*, 29, no. 1 (2013): 33–39, https://foodpsy-
chology.cornell.edu/research/you-taste-what-you-see-do
-organic-labels-bias-taste-perceptions.

27. Dr. Alison Armstrong, in discussion with the author,
January 2017.

28. Brian Wansink, Robert Kent, and Stephen Hoch, "An
Anchoring and Adjustment Model of Purchase Quantity
Decisions," Abstract, *Journal of Marketing Research*, 35 (February

1998): 71–81, http://foodpsychology.cornell.edu/research/anchoring-and-adjustment-model-purchase-quantity-decisions.

29. Sam K. Hui, Eric T. Bradlow, and Peter S. Fader, "Testing Behavioral Hypotheses Using an Integrated Model of Grocery Store Shopping Path and Purchase Behavior," Abstract, *Journal of Consumer Research*, 36, no. 3 (October 2009): 478–493, http://www.jstor.org/stable/10.1086/599046.

30. Chris Weller, "The Psychology of Shopping: How Grocery Stores Make Rational Spending Nearly Impossible," *Medical Daily*, November 21, 2013, http://www.medicaldaily.com/psychology-shopping-how-grocery-stores-make-rational-spending-nearly-impossible-263393.

31. Rupp, "Surviving the Sneaky Psychology."

Chapter 6

1. Johns Hopkins University Bloomberg School of Public Health, "Home Cooking a Main Ingredient in Healthier Diet, Study Shows," ScienceDaily, November 17, 2014, https://www.sciencedaily.com/releases/2014/11/141117084711.htm.

2. Brian Wansink, James M. Painter, and Koert van Ittersum, "Descriptive Menu Labels Effect on Sales," Abstract, *The Cornell Hotel and Restaurant Administrative Quarterly*, 42, no. 6 (2001): 68–72. http://www.sciencedirect.com/science/article/pii/S0010880401810119.

3. Eleanor Harding, "Your Mum's Sunday Roast or Grandmother's Apple Pie? A Meal Made with Love Really

DOES Taste Better," *Daily Mail*, updated January 19, 2012, http://www.dailymail.co.uk/news/article-2089181/A-meal-love-really-DOES-taste-better.html. To download the original study, go to Kurt Gray, "The Power of Good Intentions: Perceived Benevolence Soothes Pain, Increases Pleasure, and Improves Taste," Abstract, *Social Psychological and Personality Science*, 3, no. 5 (September 1, 2012): 639–645, https://doi.org/10.1177/1948550611433470.

4. Harriet Brown, "Go with Your Gut," *The New York Times*, February 20, 2006, http://www.nytimes.com/2006/02/20/opinion/go-with-your-gut.html?mcubz=0.

5. Gray, "The Power of Good Intentions."

6. Dan Charnas, "For a More Ordered Life, Organize Like a Chef," *The Salt* (blog), *Morning Edition*, NPR, Boise State Public Radio, August 11, 2014, http://www.npr.org/sections/thesalt/2014/08/11/338850091/for-a-more-ordered-life-organize-like-a-chef.

7. Aubrey, "A Cluttered Kitchen."

8. Brian Wansink, Andrew Hanks, and Kirsikka Kaipainen, "Slim by Design: Kitchen Counter Correlates of Obesity," Abstract, *Health Education and Behavior*, 43, no. 5 (October 2016): 552–558, doi:10.1177/1090198115610571.

9. Ata Jami, "Healthy Reflections: The Influence of Mirror Induced Self-Awareness on Taste Perceptions," *Journal of the Association for Consumer Research*, 1 no. 1, published ahead of print, September 20, 2015, https://ssrn.com/abstract=2689382.

10. Linda Varone (Feng Shui Expert), in discussion with the author, November 2016.

11. C. Houston-Price et al., "Picture Book Exposure Elicits Positive Visual Preferences in Toddlers," *Journal of Experimental Child Psychology*, 104 (2009): 89–104, https://www.ncbi.nlm.nih.gov/pubmed/19427645.

12. Koert van Ittersum and Brian Wansink, "Plate Size and Color Suggestibility: The Delboeuf Illusion's Bias on Serving and Eating Behavior," *Journal of Consumer Research*, 39, no. 2 (August 1, 2012): 215–228, https://academic.oup.com/jcr/article/39/2/215/1795747/Plate-Size-and-Color-Suggestibility-The-Delboeuf.

13. Jessica Firger, "Brain Food: How Neurogastronomy Will Soon Alter Your Perception of Flavor," *Newsweek*, April 27, 2016, http://www.newsweek.com/2016/05/06/neurogastronomy-taste-deprivation-smell-loss-palatable-food-452819.html.

14. James Temperton, "Heavy Cutlery Makes Food Taste Better," *Wired*, July 23, 2015, http://www.wired.co.uk/article/heavy-cutlery-food-taste-better.

15. Charles Michel, Carlos Velasco, and Charles Spence, "Cutlery Matters: Heavy Cutlery Enhances Diners' Enjoyment of the Food Served in a Realistic Dining Environment," BioMed Central, *Flavour Journal*, 4, no. 26 (July 23, 2015), https://doi.org/10.1186/s13411-015-0036-y.

16. Laura Blue, "Using a Big Fork May Help You Eat Less," *Time*, July 15, 2011, http://healthland.time.com/2011/07/15/using-a-big-fork-may-help-you-eat-less/.

17. Brian Wansink and Koert van Ittersum, "Bottoms Up! The Influence of Elongation and Pouring on Consumption Volume," Abstract, *Journal of Consumer Research*, 30, no. 3 (2003): 455–463. https://academic.oup.com/jcr/

article-abstract/30/3/455/1790637/Bottoms-Up-The-Influence-
of-Elongation-on-Pouring?redirectedFrom
=fulltext.

18. Kathleen D. Vohs et al., "Rituals Enhance Consumption,"
    Psychological Science, 24, no. 9 (September 1, 2013): 1714–1721,
    https://doi.org/10.1177/0956797613478949.

Chapter 7

1. Maria Konnikova, "Altered Tastes," *New Republic,*
   February 15, 2016, https://newrepublic.com/article/128899/
   man-will-transform-eat.

2. Konnikova, "Altered Tastes."

3. Ty Wagoner, "Flavor: It's All in Your Head!," *Science
   Meets Food,* January 17, 2017, http://sciencemeetsfood.org/
   flavor-its-all-in-your-head/.

4. Whitney Filloon, "How Fine Dining Chef Heston
   Blumenthal Could Change Mass Marketed
   Food for the Better," *Eater,* February 19, 2016,
   https://www.eater.com/2016/2/19/11059048/
   heston-blumenthal-profile-cooking-neurogastronomy.

5. Jozef Youssef, "Defining Gastrophysics," Kitchen Theory,
   February 17, 2016, https://www.kitchen-theory.com/
   defining-gastrophysics-1/.

6. Youssef, "Defining Gastrophysics."

7. "Chivas Ultimate Cask Collection Senseploration,"
   Kitchen Theory, accessed June 1, 2017, https://

www.kitchen-theory.com/portfolio-item/
chivas-ultimate-cask-collection-senseploration/.

8. *Food Science and Technology*, "Enhancing the Experience through Smell," January 6, 2016, http://www.fstjournal.org/features/30-2/olfactory-augmentation.

9. Janice Wang (Graduate Student in Charles Spence's Lab), in discussion with the author, February 2017.

10. Anne-Sylvie Crisinel et al., "A Bittersweet Symphony: Systematically Modulating the Taste of Food by Changing the Sonic Properties of the Soundtrack Playing in the Background," Abstract, *Food Quality and Preference*, 24, no. 1 (April 2012): 201–204, https://doi.org/10.1016/j.foodqual.2011.08.009.

11. Layla Eplett, "The Sound (and Taste) of Music," *Scientific American*, December 9, 2014, https://blogs.scientificamerican.com/food-matters/the-sound-and-taste-of-music/.

12. Eplett, "The Sound (and Taste) of Music."

13. Janice Wang, discussion.

14. Charles Spence, "Noise and Its Impact on the Perception of Food and Drink," BioMed Central, *Flavour Journal*, 3, no. 9 (November 20, 2014), https://flavourjournal.biomedcentral.com/articles/10.1186/2044-7248-3-9.

15. Lisa Ryan, "Want to Know the Key to Weight Loss? Listen Up! People Eat Less If They're More Aware of the 'Crunch Effect'—How Loud They Chew Their Food," *Daily Mail*, March 16, 2016, http://www.dailymail.co.uk/health/article-3495332/Want-know-key-weight-loss-LISTEN-People-eat-aware-crunch-effect-loud-chew-food.html.

Notes

16. Massimiliano Zampini and Charles Spence, "The Role of Auditory Cues in Modulating the Perceived Crispness and Staleness of Potato Chips," *Journal of Sensory Studies*, 19 (October 2004): 347–363, doi:10.1111/j.1745-459x.2004.080403.x.

17. Emily Sohn, "Taste Buds and 'Tude: The Food and Mood Link," *Los Angeles Times*, September 6, 2012, http://articles.latimes.com/2012/sep/06/health/la-he-food-morals-20120818.

18. Sohn, "Taste Buds and 'Tude."

19. Jane Ogden, Eirini Oikonomou, and Georgina Alemany, "Distraction, Restrained Eating and Disinhibition: An Experimental Study of Food Intake and the Impact of 'Eating on the Go,'" Abstract, *Journal of Health Psychology*, 22, no. 1 (January 1, 2017): 39–50, https://doi.org/10.1177/1359105315595119.

20. N. I. Larson et al., "Making Time for Meals: Meal Structure and Associations with Dietary Intake in Young Adults," Abstract, *Journal of American Diet Association*, 109, no. 1 (January 2009): 72–79, https://www.ncbi.nlm.nih.gov/pubmed/19103325.

21. Amy Fleming, "The Joys of Grazing," *The Guardian*, September 30, 2014, https://www.theguardian.com/lifeandstyle/wordofmouth/2014/sep/30/grazing-underrated-way-to-eat.

22. Sarah Knapton, "Why Eating Breakfast on the Go Really Does Lead to Weight Gain," *The Telegraph*, August 20, 2015, http://www.telegraph.co.uk/news/science/science-news/11812141/Why-eating-breakfast-on-the-go-helps-pile-on-the-pounds.html.

23. Eric Robinson et al., "Eating Attentively: A Systematic Review and Meta-Analysis of the Effect of Food Intake Memory and Awareness on Eating," Abstract, *The American Journal of Clinical Nutrition*, 97, no. 4 (April 2013): 728–742, http://ajcn.nutrition.org/content/early/2013/02/25/ajcn.112.045245.abstract.

24. American Mindfulness Research Association, "Mindful Attention Helps Regulate Amount of Food Consumed," April 15, 2016, https://goamra.org/mindful-attention-helps-regulate-amount-food-consumed/.

25. Spence, "Noise and Its Impact."

26. C. S. Yang, M. J. Lee, and L. Chen, "Human Salivary Tea Catechin Levels and Catechin Esterase Activities: Implication in Human Cancer Prevention Studies," Abstract, *Cancer Epidemiology, Biomarkers and Prevention*, 8, no. 1 (January 1999): 83–89, https://www.ncbi.nlm.nih.gov/pubmed/9950244.

27. Brian St. Pierre, "All About Eating Slowly," Precision Nutrition, May 1, 2017, http://www.precisionnutrition.com/all-about-slow-eating.

28. St. Pierre, "All About Eating Slowly."

29. Alexander Kokkinos et al., "Eating Slowly Increases the Postprandial Response of the Anorexigenic Gut Hormones, Peptide YY and Glucagon-Like Peptide-1," *The Journal of Clinical Endocrinology and Metabolism*, 95, no. 1, (January 1, 2010): 333–337, https://doi.org/10.1210/jc.2009-1018.

30. Kokkinos et al., "Eating Slowly."

31. "Chewing More May Increase Satiety but Did Not Reduce

Food Intake at Next Meal," EUFIC, September 17, 2013, http://www.eufic.org/en/healthy-living/article/chewing-more-may-increase-satiety-but-did-not-reduce-food-intake-at-next-me.

32. J. H. Hollis and Y. Zhu, "Increasing the Number of Chews Before Swallowing Reduces Meal Size in Normal-Weight, Overweight, and Obese Adults," Abstract, *Journal of the Academy of Nutrition and Dietetics*, 114, no. 6 (June 2014): 926–931, https://www.ncbi.nlm.nih.gov/pubmed/24215801.

33. Institute of Food Technologists, "Chew More to Retain More Energy," *Science Daily*, July 15, 2013, www.science-daily.com/releases/2013/07/130715134643.htm.

34. Traci Pedersen, "Focus on Eating Pleasure Can Lead to Smaller Portions," Psych Central, October 22, 2016, https://psychcentral.com/news/2016/10/22/focus-on-eating-pleasure-can-lead-to-smaller-portions/111502.html.

35. Ram Dass, quote, Quotes, accessed September 8, 2017, http://www.quotes.net/quote/12336.

Appendix A

1. Swami Rama, "The Real Meaning of Meditation," *Yoga International*, June 3, 2013, https://yogainternational.com/article/view/the-real-meaning-of-meditation.

2. Herbert Benson, quote on Benson's official website, RelaxationResponse.org, accessed March 1, 2017, http://www.relaxationresponse.org/.

About the Author

Heather Sears is a busy chick, award winning marketing executive, and happy mom who likes to eat well and live mindfully. She lives in Boston with her husband and son where she runs an e-commerce and consulting business. Prior to founding her company, Kensho Kitchen, Heather was Vice President, Marketing for a media company where she led all aspects of marketing in a division with $150 million in revenue. In addition to other pursuits, she volunteers as a meditation and mindfulness teacher and enjoys tennis and cooking. Heather has a BA with high honors in Asian Studies and Communications from the University of Michigan and an MBA from the Kellogg Graduate School of Management at Northwestern University. *Mind to Mouth* is her first book.

Connect with her and find additional content on mindful consumption at www.heather-sears.com.

Made in the USA
Middletown, DE
25 November 2017